GOODBYE, CANCER
I FOUGHT AND WON

Ekaterina Carlos Gersten

May 2021

CONTENT

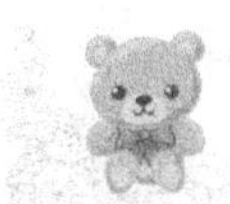
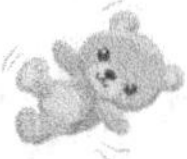
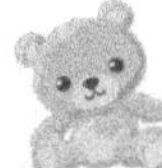
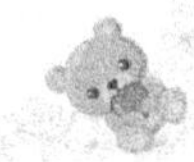

Thanks

If it weren't for my mommy, neither this book nor I would exist. Thanks to my dear mommy for helping me remember the moments we survived together. I felt everything again, like my emotions, worries, fear, sadness, pain, love, tears going back to the past to be able to write this book. Some moments in the past are painful memories, better not even remember them. Every memory made me cry before I could write it down. Then I calmed down and continued writing, returning to the body of a six-year-old girl, which was me.

I want to thank my brothers Pavel and Klim for supporting me all the time, especially in the hardest moments of my life, trying to calm me down, making jokes about the boys at school, helping me feel good for a while. His words and emotions made me feel so much better. When Pavel went to the United States and I stayed with Klim, he protected me at school, not being understood by my classmates who rejected me in their circuit of friends.

To write my book I had to interview my relatives, my mommy, my grandmother, my daddy, Pavel, Klim, my uncle Ilusha, my aunt Liubasha and my cousins Adelina and Melani to reconstruct my childhood memories. Without them I could not remember my story in detail.

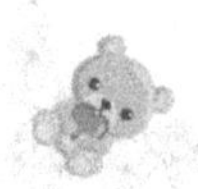 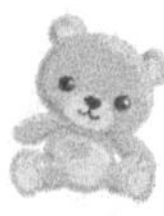 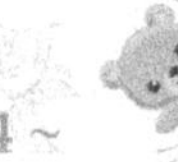 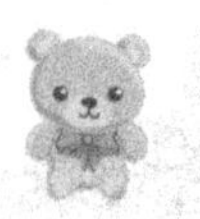

Thanks to my dad for all his help and love.

Thanks to my dolls that at that time of my childhood were like part of my family, in such a way that they generated positive energy for me by having to take care of them so that they did not get sick, for that I had to be very strong.

Thanks to the doctors who treated me in the best possible way.

Thanks to my teacher Brian McDermott for protecting me and making me feel good in his class.

Thanks to the Universe for opening its doors to infinity and allowing me to escape from the hands of the wolf, to become my friend just in time and to teach me not to be afraid of him.

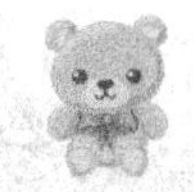 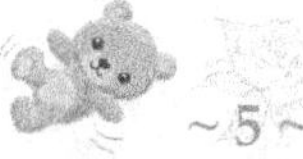 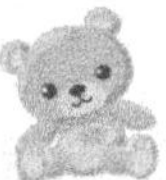 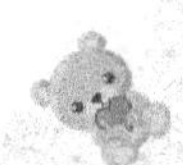

Introduction

I had to face a terrible disease that almost ended my life when I was only six years old. My mommy's effort to find alternatives to save me, along with the unconditional love of my family, who never left me alone, is what made it possible for me to tell you my story from top to bottom.

As children, we don't know much about life, or about the extremes we go through. Kids understand their feelings, if they're hurt or uncomfortable, wishing it could be possible to play and run like others... it fills us with sadness to see that for some reason we can't do normal things, ignoring the seriousness of what we're dealing with. That's our loved ones' job, to take care of their "adult stuff" to make us feel better.

Now that I'm a young girl, I can see things more clearly, and talk about the negative effect that society, some people pressure, and the modern lifestyle can have on our lives. I want to share with everyone how beautiful a life in harmony and love is, combined with all the good that nature gives us and a healthy community provides.

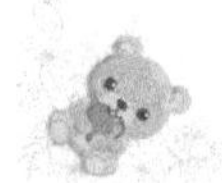 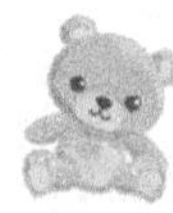 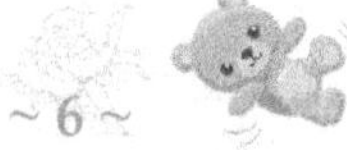 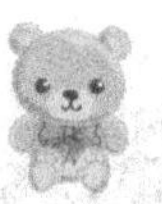

The majority of this book is written by my child self, with her feelings, experiences and emotions, which were not so easy to tell. My mommy and I thought of a way to tell you this same story, from two very different angles, which might be similar, but very different from each other as well. A book told by the mommy, and another one told by her daughter, who is me: Katerina.

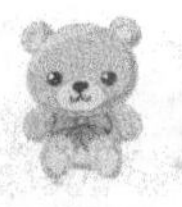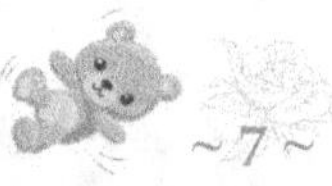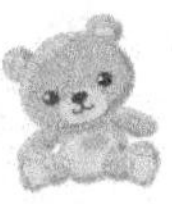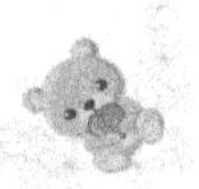

RELATING MY STORY

My Family

Hi! My name is Katerina and I'm six years old. I was born in Tarragona, but I currently live in Barcelona (Spain) with my family: my mommy, and my two older brothers. I was, and still am, the smallest of the house.

My family is wonderful and I loved them very much! My mommy's name is Liudmila, but I liked to call her "Mamita". She is super gorgeous and a smart woman who was born in Russia – an enormous country far, far away from here. I'd never been there, but my mommy told me that there was a lot of snowfall in winter. And besides, I didn't really like the cold weather, but the snow is a part of another story…I loved playing with it.

My mommy constantly showed me how much she loved me. She called me her "dochenka" – her little princess. Mamita took me everywhere, bought me Hello Kitty stuff and made my pigtails. I slept in her arms every time I had nightmares. No doubt she's the most extraordinary mom in the whole wide world!

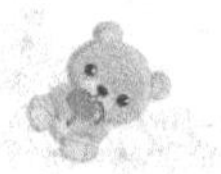 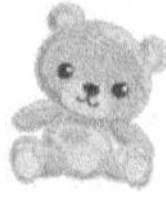 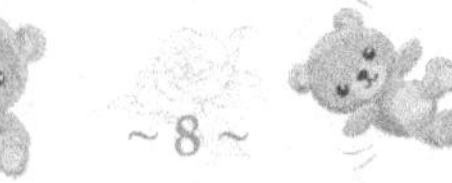 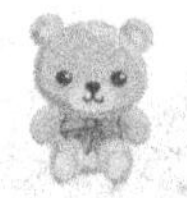

I wanted to be just like her when I grew up. I wanted to wear everything she wore – the heels, the dresses…oh! I couldn't wait to show off her beautiful necklaces that I liked so much. Her hair was so long and pretty. It always sparkled, almost like it was drenched in glitter. We had so much fun when we played beauty salon (I know how to make different hairstyles) and we were just like best friends! We had girl secrets that we didn't tell anyone. Not even the boys.

Mamita also knew how to cook the most delicious food, although, sometimes she made me drink icky juices that I didn't like at all, or eat weird insipid vegetables. I preferred the taste of pizza, but I knew she did it for my well-being because she cared for me whenever I got sick. My mommy is the most precious and gentle person, and she meant the universe to me.

Then there was Pavel, my oldest brother, who was twelve. He was my keeper when Mamita wasn't home, and took care of me anytime I got into trouble. Like the one time I knocked over a glass of water and made a mess, or when I didn't pick up my toys after playing with them. Pavel let me know I had to take care of these things, as daddy would have. I respected him as an adult and when I didn't heed his words, he reproved me just like daddy did, and I had to listen. Moreover, Pavel knew everything! It didn't matter what question I asked him because he always had an intelligent answer.

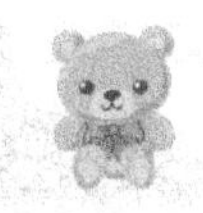 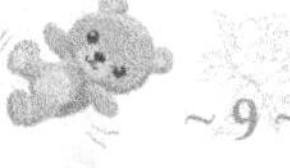 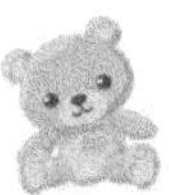 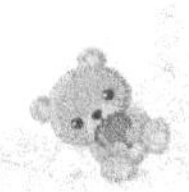

Klim, on the other hand, was ten and the middle child. Like a sandwich filling! He always played with me. Klim was a fabulous artist who made the most beautiful drawings, and liked listening to some boring music… I think it was called "classical" music, or something like that.

The two of them were my best friends on earth!

The rest of my family was incredibly awesome too!

First there was my granny. I called her "yaya" or "babulia" as we shared the same name, Katerina. She loves me so much. I often liked to think that I was a granny's girl because of how I got to cuddle with her and the goodies we baked together.

I cannot forget about auntie Liubasha, my mom's twin sister. The two of them were identical, like raindrops, yet different in their own way. I'd never gotten confused between the two of them. It might sound silly, but I've always known my mom as my mom, and my aunt as my aunt; which reminds me – Liubasha has a husband called Joan, and they are both my godparents. I'm not really sure what that meant, but I was glad they are. Oh! And they have two daughters: Adelina and Melani.

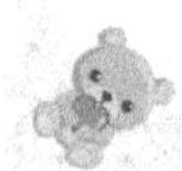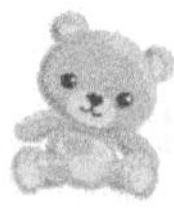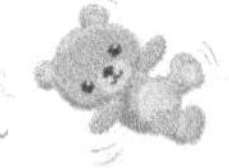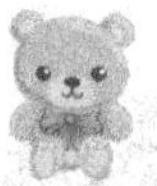

My cousin Adelina was twelve, just like my brother Pavel. She was a rhythmic gymnastics champion and performed the most amazing dances. She could jump really high, do back flips and splits in the air, or by foot. She made them look so easy and never fell over like I did. Whenever we had parties at babulia's house, we had karaoke and other contests. My cousins and I liked to perform a show when we celebrated New Year's, and Adelina and I always had some wonderful dances choreographed by Adelina. I really enjoyed it! I definitely wanted to be a gymnast like her when I grew up.

Adelina's little sister, my other cousin, Melani, was three years old. She was as tiny as the dolls she loved. Sometimes I played with her.

There was also my uncle Ilya. He was nineteen and a huge fan of races, and loved a car called the Lamborghini.

And then there was my dad, who loved me a whole lot. He didn't live with us though, but I still saw him from time to time.

The truth is, I had a lovely family!

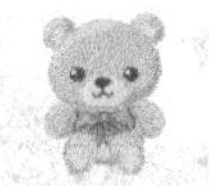 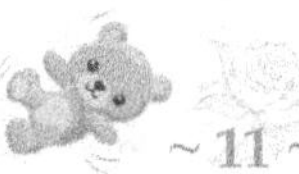 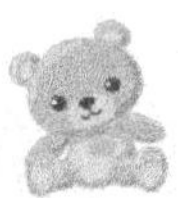 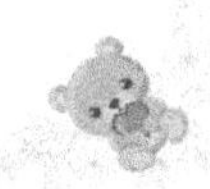

By the way, I attended the Ignasi Iglesias School in Barcelona. I was in the last cycle of pre-school and would be finishing the year in a few days. Soon, I'd be in elementary school! I was also in a rhythm gymnastics team and we practiced every day. By the end of the school year, we would be going to a championship, thanks to our two trainers who motivated us to bring out the best in us. We had to listen to them if we wanted to improve, and didn't want to make them angry

THE ASTRONAUT PICTURE

One day, mommy and daddy took me to a place with numerous doctors. It seemed my speech had some issues. They didn't always understand me, even though I spoke well and understood myself perfectly. Anyway, their concerns had them take me to a specialist – not the doctor we always went to, but a different one. The ride to his office was longer, and my parents called him a Neurologist. What an odd name, don't you think?

We arrived at a huge hospital with many different levels, giant doors, stairs, corridors, doctors and many, many sick people. That's what I liked least – their faces and their energy made me feel blue. My daddy told me that the doctors were going to take some special photos of me. They were called "astronaut photos" since they only took the photos of very brave people. It sounded like an adult concept and I liked taking pictures of astronauts, though I didn't know what they were or what they looked like, it sounded interesting.

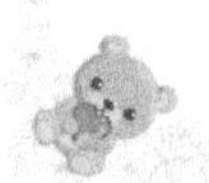
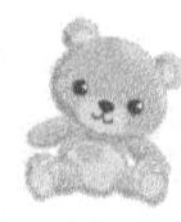
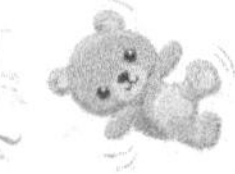
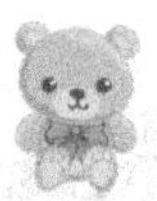

They took me to a spacious room with a huge machine that looked like a truck and had a special camera for astronauts, as my daddy told me. Since I was quite brave, they were going to take these singular photos of me. It was only later that I learned the name of the camera-truck: "Magnetic Resonance Imaging (MRI)".

A photographer – rather, a photo-doctor, who wore a white coat (I didn't even know there were doctor photographers), had me lay down on a long, uncomfortable bed. It was very hard and long, and I was suddenly terrified of falling. This bed moved in and out of the camera-truck. He placed a big helmet on my head and strapped it in place so that I wouldn't move my head. They wanted the photos to come out perfect. They told me that they were going to take thousands of photos and that it would take a while. I had to remain very calm. I didn't want the photos to come out looking ugly.

They injected a transparent liquid into my arm, assuring me that it wouldn't hurt, and that it was like a mosquito bite — I didn't really like mosquitoes. I was then taken inside the camera-truck, riding on the rolling bed, to start the session. It was scary! The tunnel was too tight! But I was very brave. I realized there were funny stickers inside the tube, and so I amused myself by looking at them.

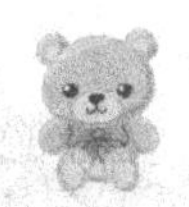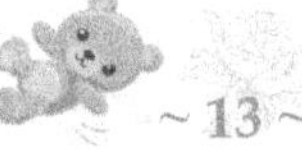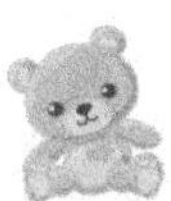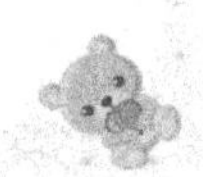

Besides, Mamita was standing right next to me with her hands on my feet, which made me feel better and my fears dissipated a little. Mamita was also given huge headphones during the session. Finally, the doctor came to see us and assured us that nothing would happen to me, and that I didn't have to be afraid.

They put on some cartoons for me so I wouldn't get bored and then they tucked me inside a blanket because I was trembling from the cold (the room felt like a freezer). They said they were only going to take pictures of my head. All the photo-doctors left the room, leaving only me, my mommy, and the astronaut machine inside. The engines started running, and the device made a rumbling sound like it was going to break. It reminded me of the "Tack! Tack! Tack!" noise my daddy made when he spiked the screws into the walls (but almost a thousand times louder). However, I was brave and ready for my modeling sessions, and that's what mattered.

I couldn't watch the cartoons very well because of the loud noise or hear anything. I was bored and tired. I wanted them to stop since the session was taking too long. I felt my baby eyes closing, and in the end, it seemed I'd fallen asleep. The noise from the machine finally stopped at some point and I woke up then. They pulled me out of the tube and took off the big helmet.

"Is my photo session over?" I asked them curiously.

"Yes queen, it's over now."

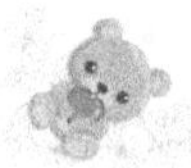 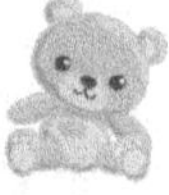 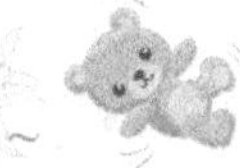 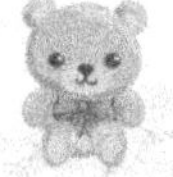

I really hoped I hadn't moved around in my sleep and that the pictures turned out pretty. They told me that I was very brave during the session and that the photos wouldn't be ready for a while, so we had to wait.

WE ARE BIG AND RESPONSIBLE

I attended a school called Ignasi Iglesias and absolutely loved it. Most of the time when we woke up early in the mornings, my mommy was not home. She had to work very hard, not to mention the university. Mami never stopped, poor thing, and was often exhausted. That was the reason why she left home very, very early and I didn't always get to see her when the sun came up. So, we had to do things on our own since we weren't babies anymore. We were quite grown up and could take care of ourselves. My brothers would wake me up and help me get dressed for school. They forced me to brush my teeth every morning and I listened to them, unless they took their eyes off me – at which point I wouldn't, and went to school without doing it.

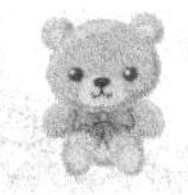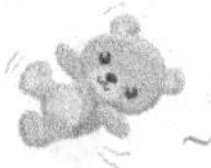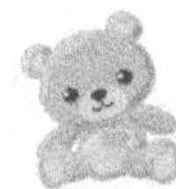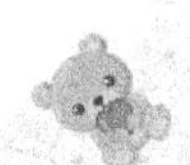

In my backpack, I always carried a snack Mamita prepared for me, a juice box, and every now and then, some fruit. Or cookies. My mommy made the most delicious sandwiches with cheese and ham. I loved sandwiches, but let me tell you a little secret of mine – they tasted better without bread. In the playground, sometimes when the teachers weren't watching me, I'd throw the bread away and eat my favorite sandwich. Yummy! I also liked donuts, but Mamita didn't buy them too often because "they have a lot of sugar and fat" even though they tasted so good! I truly enjoyed the delightful taste of sweets. Whenever my daddy came to visit, he would always buy them for me – big donuts and chocolate milk.

We lived in a very huge, new building. Mamita had taught us to always greet the neighbors, but they were very serious people.

Not everyone responded to us, and that is without the unfriendly looks they gave us. Whenever we left the house, Pavel or Klim would lock the door so that no one could break in. We all had a copy of the house key and I made sure to hide mine very well so it wouldn't get lost; mommy told me I needed it in case the boys dropped theirs or misplaced it, so I kept a close eye on my key and continuously checked it to make sure it was in its place. She trusted me because she knew how responsible I was!

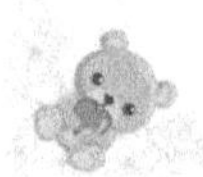
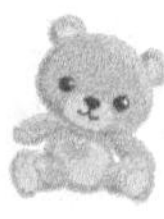
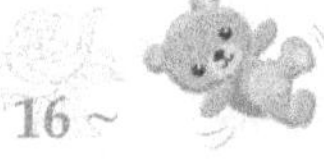
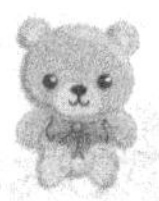

Then, we went down the stairs, which is something I didn't like since there were so many of them! Besides, Pavel and Klim usually ended up running down fast and I was always left behind. I was afraid to be left alone there so if the boys disappeared, I cried out in fear. Even though the building had a huge elevator (in fact, it had two), Mamita didn't let us use them without being accompanied by an adult. She told us that it could occasionally stop working and we could end up trapped inside without being able to get out. An adult might know what to do in that situation, but not a child. Nevertheless, sometimes we got on the elevator without letting mama know.

My brothers used to tell me, "Katerina, don't say anything to mommy or she'll get mad at us."

And, of course, since I didn't like using the stairs and I didn't want Mamita to get mad either, I didn't tell her anything about it. I liked going down in the elevator and since my brothers were there by my side, I didn't have to be alone. So we really did a good job of keeping the secret among the three of us.

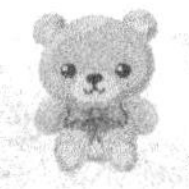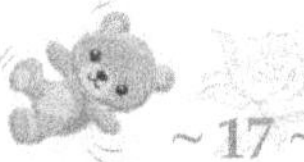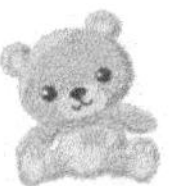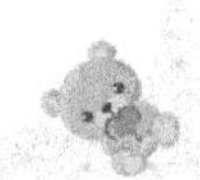

Once we went out onto the streets, we had to cross the road. To me, this was the most complicated part. We had to wait for the light to change colors and display a miniature green person walking. Mamita warned us that even if the light had the green person on it, we were not supposed to cross alone without adults because we were small and drivers might not see us and run us over. We had to always wait for an adult to come along. At times, we had to wait for two or three light changes until someone came along, and when someone arrived, we would cross with that person. We didn't say anything, but we felt safer having an adult nearby, just like Mami told us.

Right after crossing the traffic light was the long, straight walk to the school. This path lay wedged between the road and a high wall. Mom told us to always walk by the fence and never near the highway. Pavel and Klim were to walk on each side of me. We weren't supposed to drop hands until we reached the school. I felt so safe flanked by my two brothers on both sides. I knew nothing would happen to me because my brothers were big – bigger than me, at least.

Mamita also advised us that if a car stopped nearby and an adult called out to us, we were not to get close to them at all. Never, ever, ever! They could be bad, or even dangerous people! So, every time we walked down that path, I always kept an eye out for any cars that might stop next to us.

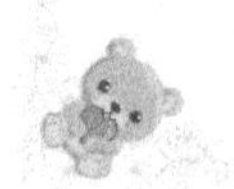 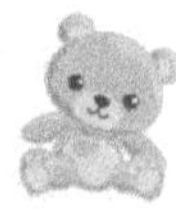 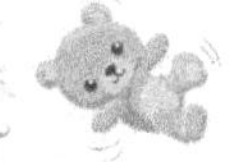 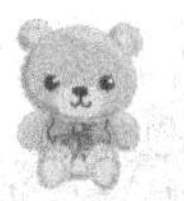

We continued on our way until we reached another narrow street.

We had to look very carefully to the right and left, and again to the right, before crossing (as mommy had taught us) the street which was right next to the school. She told us that the cars didn't always stop, and therefore, reminded us to be cautious each time we crossed. We had to wait until there were no cars around.

This was a tradition that we'd been following this since I was four years old, and I knew very well what we had to do, by then.

I remember, one time, when Klim was almost run over by a crazy driver. We were walking with my mom across a pedestrian crossing that was close to our house. We were all walking together and were almost at the middle of the street, which was quite wide. Suddenly, we saw a car approaching us at full speed and stopped immediately out of fear. But Klim, who was ahead of us, hopping like a bunny in a straight line, hadn't seen us, nor did he see the car.

Mami screamed in fright. "STOP, KLIM, STOP!"

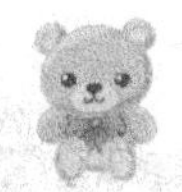 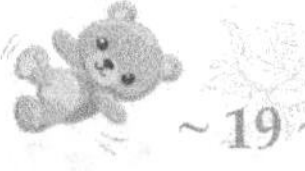 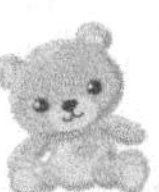 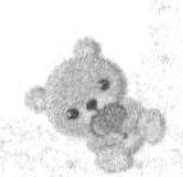

But Klim was in the middle of a jump and didn't hear Mami. The car came so fast that it almost ran over him. Quickly, Klim jumped backwards at the same moment that the crazy car passed in front of our faces, braking and squealing as the wheels skid down the path. It passed so close I felt it almost touching my nose. The car was only able to brake completely when it reached the bus stop, which was further away from the crosswalk. The driver was going so fast he couldn't get the car to stop on time.

Mommy was so scared she started crying, as did I. I cried any time I saw Mamita in tears. The people who had been crossing, also stopped and exclaimed in terror, "Who drives so madly around the city where a number of people and children are walking?"

Some of them insulted the driver using swear words that I could not repeat. Being a child, I was not to repeat such terrible words. I'm not sure the crazy driver heard them since he was inside his car and left in a hurry. The others clamoured around Klim and asked him if he was okay. My mommy, dropping the bags on the floor, started crying in panic and pulled Klim into a tight hug. I don't think he was as scared because he didn't seem to understand what was going on, for it had all happened so fast. Thank God, Klim was okay! What would I do with only one brother?

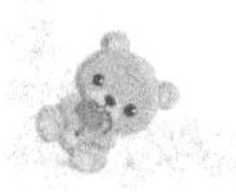 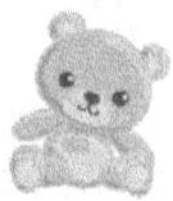 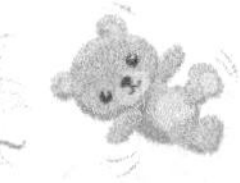 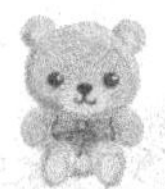

So, since then, the rule of crossing the street was well established and understood and we made sure never to break it. We knew there were many crazy drivers on the street.

Some days, Pilar, a friend of my mom's, picked us up by car and took us to school, especially when the weather was very cold or it rained. Her daughter, Paula, was in the same class as I, and we were friends who would talk from time to time. On some days, when Mami didn't have early classes at the university or a different schedule at her job, she took us to school.

We had memorized all the rules well, and also knew our home address, along with Mami's phone number! Mamita sometimes made us complete her sentences to see who answered first. She did it so many times that it was impossible to forget the right information.

I HAVE A "LITTLE NUT" IN MY HEAD

There were only a few days of school left and the summer holidays were well around the corner. At the end of the year, we usually had a performance at the Rhythmic Gymnastics School which I attended every day. Since it was my last year in the children's course, I knew I'd be graduating soon and would be joining the elementary school. I felt all grown up! I would be studying in a bigger building close to my brothers and wouldn't be with kids anymore!

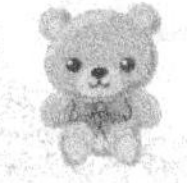 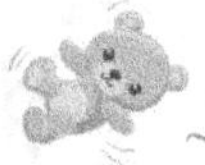 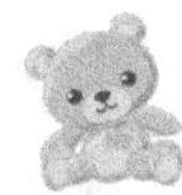 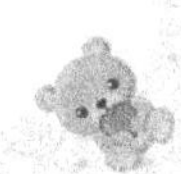

The astronaut pictures were finally ready and we had to get them from the hospital. I had to miss school for a day because of it. When we arrived there, we had to wait for the doctor to see us. There was a line with daddies, mommies and their kids waiting, like in a supermarket.

In the meantime, I played with the other children in the playground next to the doctor's office. Finally, my parents were called inside and the nurses took me to another, smaller, playroom. I had to wait there for mommy and daddy.

"I want to go with my mommy. I don't know why they won't let me go with them."

The doctor told me, "The nurses are going to show you something fun and you're going to like it. There are no children in this room – just me and the ladies in white. I usually have a good time with them, and they like playing with me and teaching me a fun board game. It's something about building a tower and taking out the pieces one by one… but carefully! I can't let the tower fall. Then we draw funny faces, and usually laugh a lot."

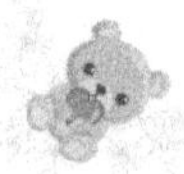
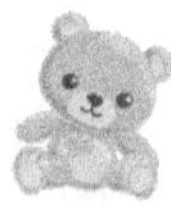
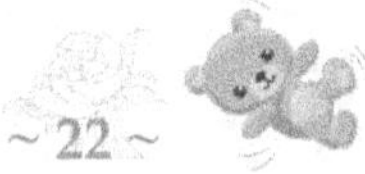
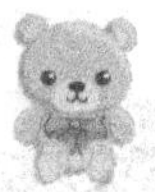

When they took me to the doctor's office, he asked me to do quite a few things like walk in a straight line, had me close my eyes and then touch the tip of my nose with my fingers, he gently tapped my knees with a tiny hammer that blew off my leg and I almost smacked his face with it. He also tickled my foot, and asked me to try some balancing exercises that went wrong and caused me to fall down.

Then the doctor told me, "Katerina, I saw your pictures and you turned out very well."

He showed me some pictures but I didn't understand... ANYTHING!

Mami explained to me, "The pictures are from the inside of your head, princess. Only doctors can understand them. You can't see your face, but he said he really liked the way you came out. You were brilliant at the photoshoot."

"Okay," I answered without really understanding what they meant. 'Thank God the doctor likes them,' I thought to myself.

We went home and I returned to school, as usual.

A few days later mommy told me, "Sweetie, do you remember the astronaut pictures we took of you, the ones the doctor liked?"

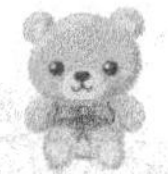 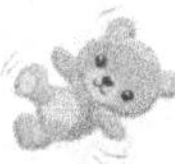 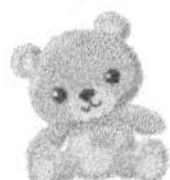 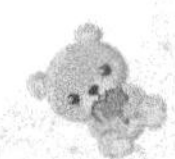

"Yes, Mamita."

"In those photos the doctor found something in your little head that shouldn't be there."

"What is it, Mami?" I asked her curiously.

"This little thing he found is a ball that's inside your head and is the size of a nut," she tried to explain.

"I have a nut... in my head, Mami?" I asked again, completely confused at her explanation.

"It's not a nut, but something like a nut. It's a little ball called a tumor. And it doesn't let you run very fast."

"What a strange name for that nut, a tumor..." I answered, "it sounds like a boy's name."

My mommy went on, "This little ball squeezes the inside of your head where the brain is. We need your brain to think, and that's the reason we have to take care of it."

"Ah. Yes, Mami?"

"Yes, princess, that's right. The doctors are thinking about what to do so that it's not in your head anymore."

Then my mommy asked me, "How well do your eyes see, Katerina? Is it good or blurry?

"What does blurry mean, Mamita?"

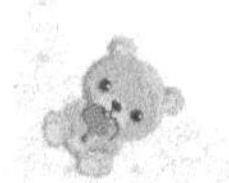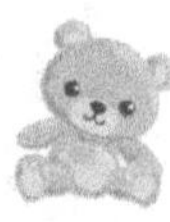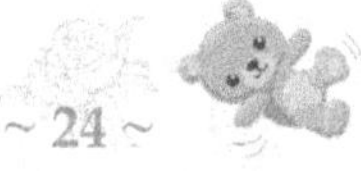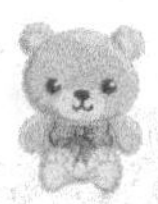

"It means… not clear, like twice the same image, it's called seeing double."

"Sometimes I see two Pavels, sometimes it's like a fog and I can't see very clearly…I get dizzy."

"All right, dóchenka, let's see what the doctors have to say."

We went back to the same hospital almost a thousand times for more and more tests, tests, more tests, and other astronaut photos. It was always the same routine… so boring!

THEY WANT TO TAKE THE "NUT" OUT OF MY HEAD

It was a quiet weekend and there was no school to attend. My whole family came to visit our home: babulia, Ilya (who we usually called Ilusha), Liubasha and my two cousins, Melani and Adelina. I really liked playing with them. My aunt's family lived close to us, but babulia and Ilusha lived in another city, a little further away.

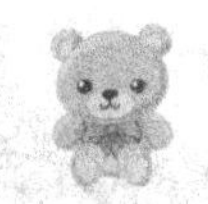
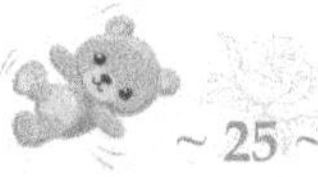
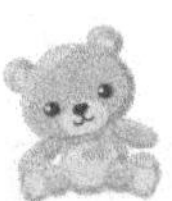
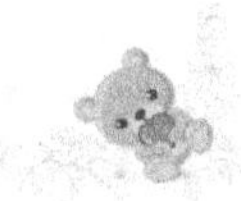

I liked it when my granny visited us because it was always like a party – she would prepare tasty meals, like pirozhki (which is a kind of Russian bun) filled with carrots, potatoes, minced meat, or cabbage; the ones stuffed with carrots were my favorite. Another nice dish was the pelmeni (these were similar to raviolis, but Russian) stuffed with cabbage or minced meat with a sauce called smetana (in Spain, it was similar to the greek yogurt that Mami bought sometimes, but tasted better) which was also very, very delicious. We took out the long table and ate together. I had a lot of fun at these meetings with my cousins. After everyone returned to their houses, we brushed our teeth and went to sleep.

The next day, Mamita wanted to tell me something. "Dóchenka, do you remember that little nut the doctor found in your head?"

"Yes, Mami, I remember. Is it still in my head? Isn't it gone?" I asked her.

"Yes, my princess, it is still there. Actually, it seems that the ball doesn't disappear… so we have to help it out. The doctors want to do something. Get it out of there, probably." I still didn't understand what she meant.

The next day, as we were talking again, Mamita told me, "Do you remember, honey, we talked about that little nut you have in your head, that the doctors want to get rid of?"

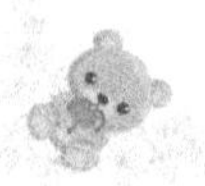 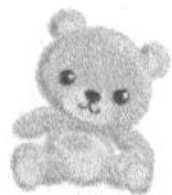 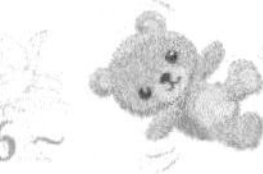 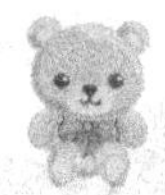

"Get rid of it, Mamita? But how? I still don't understand."

"The doctors want to do it so they can heal you, baby," my mommy continued.

"I don't really understand what you're saying, Mami… something about the nut with a boyish name."

"The doctors want to do something special, my princess. Something called 'surgery'. It will help you get better."

Again, I wished I could understand all these terms she was talking about.

Another day, at breakfast, I asked her again, "What's a surgery, Mami?"

"Mmm, how do I explain it.. A surgery is when the doctors make a small cut and then sew it back up… yes! Like a seam."

"A seam… what is that?"

"Imagine someone is going to make you a dress, the prettiest one! When that person cuts the fabric with scissors and then sews it using a thread and needle, that's how a dress is made. That cutting and sewing together make "a seam". But when they do the same thing to a person, it's called a surgery."

I listened carefully without understanding it completely. I understood the logic about the dress but not how it applied to the person.

"A seam? What a strange name…" I answered.

My mommy continued, "When they cut and sew a body part, it's called a surgery or an operation. However, in a surgery, first they make the cut, and then they take out the thing that bothers you, or what shouldn't be there. Then they sew it back up."

"Do they want to cut something out of me, Mommy?"

"Something like that."

"I don't want it Mami!" I told her.

"Don't worry, princess, everything will be fine," she soothed and calmed me down.

The next day, I asked her again, "Do bodies get cut? How do you cut your body, mommy? Is it like a wound, like when I fall down?"

"That's how it is, honey. It's similar, but when you fall down, the skin cuts itself from the fall. When we put a bandage on it and it heals itself, that cut is called a wound; but when the doctors want to do it, that's called a surgery. That's what the doctors want to do: they make a small cut, and take the "nut" out so you'll feel better."

"What? They want to cut my head off, Mamita? I don't want to be cut, Mami, I don't want to! That hurts, Mami, I don't want to! I don't want to!" I screamed and started to cry.

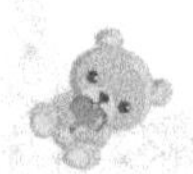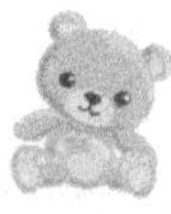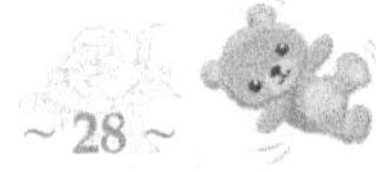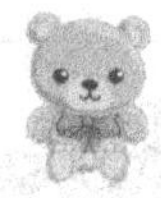

My mommy hugged me, caressed my hair and gave me kisses to calm me down again. She held me close and I felt safe since I trusted her.

"You won't really feel anything, baby. The doctors are good. Firstly, they give you medicine and you fall asleep. While you sleep, they would do their job and you wouldn't even notice."

"Not at all, Mamita?"

"Not at all. When you wake up, everything will be done. Your head will hurt a bit, at first, but the doctors will give you some magic pills so that it won't hurt and you'll start to recover quickly. But don't worry, there are still many days left."

Everything that Mamita was telling me sounded absolutely awful. I didn't want to be cut by anyone.

My mommy wanted me to understand better and said, "I'm going to tell you my story, dochenka. When I was a kid, I had a surgery too."

"Ah, yes Mami? Where?"

"In the tummy."

"Why mommy? Did you have a little "nut" too?"

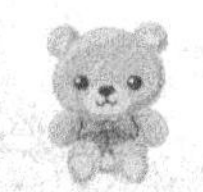 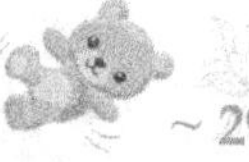 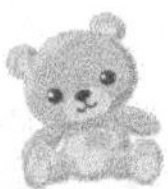 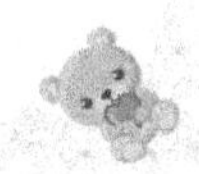

"I had a tiny bubble called appendicitis; a little thing that made my tummy hurt. You can't see the scar too clearly now because it's been so many years."

"Appendi... what?"

"Appendicitis." Mommy pulled up her shirt to show me her little cut on her tummy.

"Are you hurt, Mamita?"

"No, baby, I'm not."

"And did it hurt when you had the surgery?"

"No, I didn't feel anything, sweetheart, because I was asleep. When I woke up, it hurt a little, but then they gave me an injection to sleep and everything was over. I didn't understand anything then. I was twelve years old. I was a child, like you."

"Is that also called a sur-ge-ry, mommy?" I asked her, lightly touching her tummy.

"Exactly, little princess."

"And... Why did they cut you, Mamita?"

"Because an organ was ill and the doctors healed it. Now, I'm fine. If they hadn't done it, I could have died."

I looked up at my mommy and told her, "I don't want to die, Mamita, but I don't want to have a surgery either."

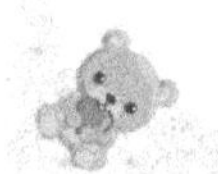 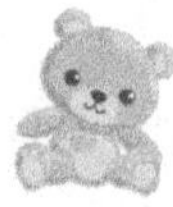 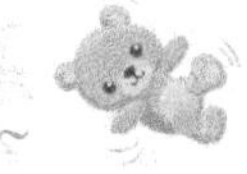 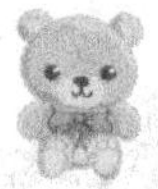

"I know, honey. No one wants you to. The doctors are going to do it very carefully and quickly to free you from that little 'nut'."

"I won't feel anything, like you, Mamita, right? Nothing at all?"

"Nothing at all, baby."

"They're going to give me some medicine so I'll sleep and not feel anything, right, Mamita?"

"That's right, baby...that's right."

I trusted my mommy and wasn't afraid after she reassured me everything would be fine. If my mommy could do it, I could, too.

Another day, my mommy told me, "You know princess, about the surgery we talked about, since they want to do it soon, we need to make a special preparation. The doctors say that you need to cut your hair."

"Cut? No, Mami! I don't want to cut my hair. I'm not a boy, why do I have to cut my hair?" I asked mommy, crying.

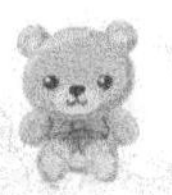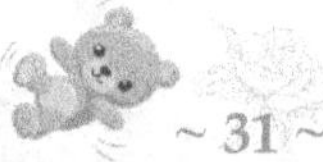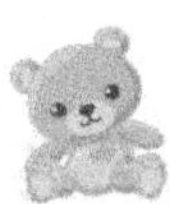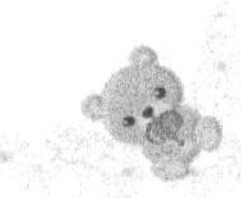

She kept her sweet voice while hugging me, "The doctors have to cut your hair so they can take the "nut" out. They say that if you don't cut your hair, it can get into the wound and that could be bad for your healing process. We want it to heal, don't we, honey?" she asked me. "We don't want anything bad to happen, right?"

"Yes, Mami, but I don't want my hair cut."

"I know, dochenka, but it's the rules. Otherwise the doctors won't get their job done."

Then, we waited for that day... My mommy told me it would be soon. I didn't know if I was scared or not, but I did know it couldn't be very good if they had to cut my hair like a boy.

I'M BALD

I had only a few days of school left and it seemed I would not be able to finish them since I had to go to the hospital for a few days. My classmates gave me an album with their drawings and photos, while my teachers told me goodbye lovingly, and wished me good luck. It was really sad and I wouldn't be able to attend the rhythmic gymnastics competition either, even though I'd really wanted to.

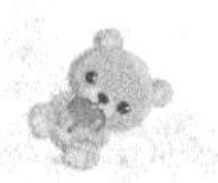
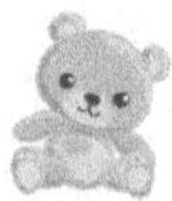
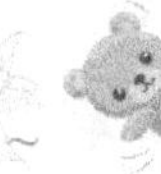
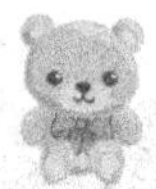

We were all packed and ready to go to the hospital, but that time it was different – it was like we were going on a trip. We packed a bag with lots of stuff, including my favorite dolls, Liudmila and Liubasha (I had two twin "daughters" whom I'd named after my mom and my aunt), and a big bear that was my best friend.

 I simply called him Oso. I also packed some of my other favorite toys, some clothes, toothpaste, drawing paper and I was ready to go to the hospital. Mami told me we'd be staying at the hospital for some days and so we had to carry enough things.

The moment we got to the hospital, the doctor took us to a room. I had to put on my pajamas and was made to lie down on my new bed. They wouldn't let me eat or drink anything but water. I was so hungry! I wanted to eat, but I was not supposed to because they kept taking blood tests.

Finally, once they were done, I went out with my mommy to the playroom and loved it since there were countless toys. Soon babulia and Liubasha arrived. My mommy told me again, "Dóchenka, do you know that tomorrow is the surgery?"

"Yes, Mommy, I know," I answered her.

"For that, we need to cut your hair," she told me softly.

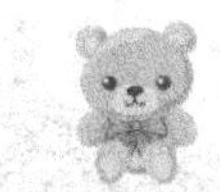
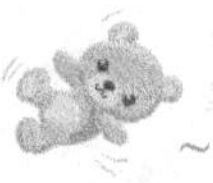
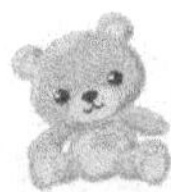
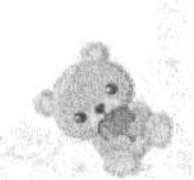

'Again with the same annoying story about the haircut!' I thought to myself. But then, mommy continued, "We can cut it later, okay? That way, at the time of the surgery, no hair will get in your wound or bother the doctors," she said, touching my hair gently.

Finally, she convinced me and I answered her, "Okay mommy, I want my hair to grow back soon!

My mommy, encouraging me, also replied, "You'll see that your hair will grow stronger, longer and prettier than ever."

"Like Rapunzel?" I asked her excitedly.

"Even better."

Daddy came to the hospital and I didn't even recognize him! He'd shaved his head like he usually shaved his face. It wasn't exactly a cut but it looked like a skating rink. I thought it was funny to see my daddy like that and I laughed.

He told me, "See, queen, you won't be alone. We'll both be the same and our hair will grow at the same time." I kept laughing. I didn't know if I agreed but I just couldn't stop laughing.

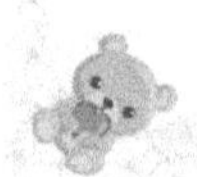 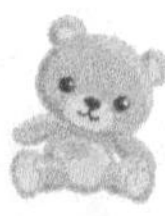 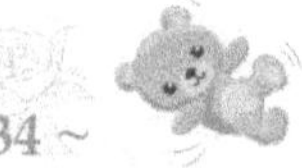 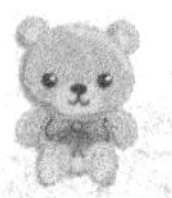

After that, I was a bit convinced, or so I thought. Besides, Daddy looked good, like a pirate who no longer scared me.

Mamita took me to the bathroom and sat me down on a chair. Liubasha, who was already there waiting, tied a huge apron around my neck.

"I'll make sure to cut your hair carefully and when it grows back, it's going to be stronger and prettier. Look at these magical scissors and shaving machines I have, they make hair grow back super-fast. You might even feel ticklish while I'm doing it."

Liubasha started cutting my hair and cheered me up saying, "I'll do it softly so you won't feel anything at all." Everyone started making jokes to make me laugh and I enjoyed it.

"Wow Katerina! You look beautiful!"

It felt like I was getting a nice haircut so I started to giggle.

"I'm done." Liubasha said after a while.

Mamita handed me a mirror and when I looked at it, I suddenly stop smiling. 'WHAT AM I SEEING? IT'S SCARY! WHO IS IN THE MIRROR? IS IT ME? I LOOK LIKE A HORRIBLE MONSTER!'

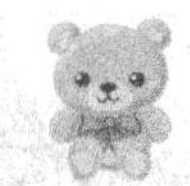 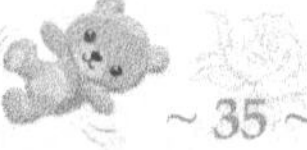 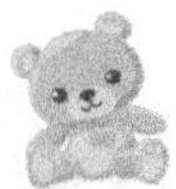 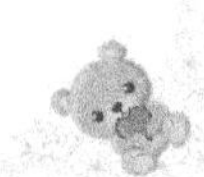

I was so scared, I started crying loudly and began screaming.

"Put my hair back on! I don't like this haircut! This is not even a haircut, I'm bald! I don't like it. I hate it! I hate it! I HATE IT!" I didn't want to talk to my aunt Liubasha anymore. I resolved never to speak to her again!

My daddy told me, "You're not alone, little queen. Look, I have the same haircut, now we're both the same, see?"

"No, no, no!" I answered crying. "You're a boy and I'm a girl! I should have long hair. I don't want to be bald! I AM UGLY!"

I couldn't stop crying and screaming. "I have no hair! I'M UGLY!" I repeated, screaming, "I'm so ugly and bald! I'm very bald and I don't like it at all! AT ALL!" I cried out loud.

"What about all those different color hair brushes I have? Now they are useless because I have no hair to brush. NOOOO! I don't want it that way! I don't want it!"

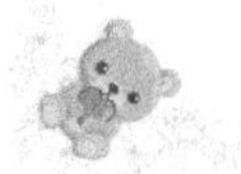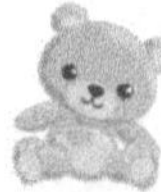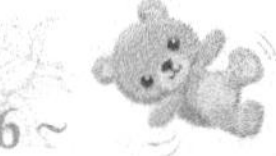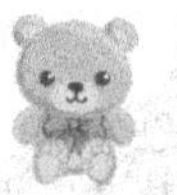

They all tried to calm me down by telling me it was only temporary, and that, soon enough, my hair would grow back even longer, stronger and prettier. But it was not helping. I just wanted my hair back at that moment. I kept wailing and I didn't know why they couldn't understand me or pay attention to me. I climbed into bed not wanting to see anyone, not even myself, thinking if I covered myself with a pillow, maybe, I could make that horrible image of myself disappear. Then, I peeked a look again in the mirror and started crying even louder. It still looked hideous. My hair still hadn't grown back.

I repeated in my head over and over again, "Ugh, how ugly I am! I want to be pretty like before! How ugly I am!" and kept crying.

Mommy had some beautiful scarves for me and covered my scary looking head with one that had a Hello Kitty print on it. At that point, I was simply too tired to cry, so she brought back the mirror and asked me, "How about now, baby?"

I warily looked at my reflection and decided it looked a bit better.

"What a gorgeous scarf you have!" My granny exclaimed. I was gradually soothed by the fact that the baldness was not visible anymore. Ugh, that was creepy!

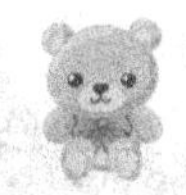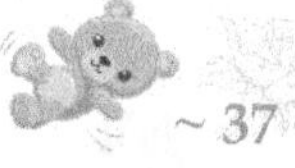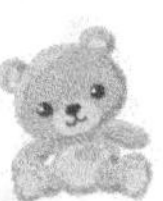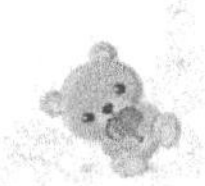

Everyone finally left, and it was just me and my mom in the room..

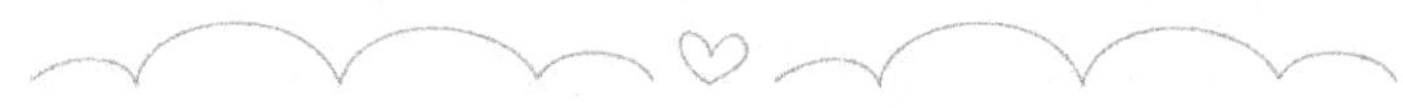

THE SURGERY

The nurses woke me up early in the morning to measure my temperature and gave me a few painful injections. I was still sleepy and wanted to go back to sleep. Babulia arrived with my dad. Another injection. I felt strange, I didn't know what or how to explain it, but I felt very strange. A nurse arrived and asked me how I felt. He said he'd be back for me with a wheeled bed. He was a funny man. He came back with a stretcher, left it in my room, and vanished again.

He came back one more time and asked me, "Are you ready to get into your Formula One, Katerina?"

"Yes! Ready," I answered.

I felt a little weird lying in the wheeled bed-car. I had nothing on and they hadn't let me wear any clothes. They just covered me with a sheet and we'd left the room making race car sounds. It seemed like the nurse knew how to drive the bed-car very well.

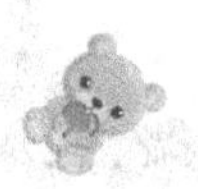 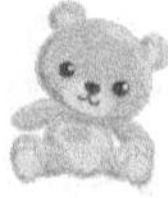 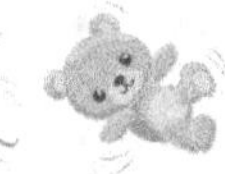 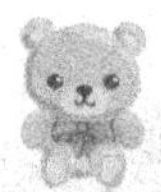

Mamita was holding my hand the entire way, so I wasn't scared. They drove me through some long halls until we got to an elevator. More halls, turn, and more halls. It was endless. When we finally reached the surgery area called the "operating room", I heard some familiar astronaut noises. Between various jokes, I got to see Mamita's eyes – she looked sad and frightened. We stood in front of a huge door. The man in a white coat who had been driving my car-bed (which I'd really liked) through the halls, left us at the entrance. Babulia and daddy stood next to me, but, to be honest, I only wanted Mami's hand and no one else's.

We were standing in front of tall white doors, and they told me they would be taking me through them, alone. It worried me terribly. It looked like something out of a horror movie. I didn't let go of my mommy's hand and thought I was safer that way.

Two more people dressed in gowns arrived, their mouths covered by something blue, and they had white shower caps on their heads. I could only see their eyes. I suddenly felt terrified and didn't feel safe anymore. I heard them tell my mom that she could say goodbye to me.

"WHAT? Goodbye? NO!" I shouted.

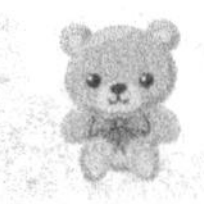
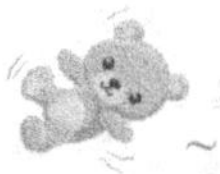
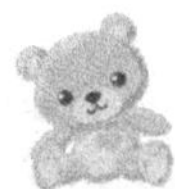
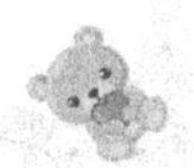

Hearing that scared me and I squeezed my mom's hand even tighter so she wouldn't let go of me. I started crying more and more, thinking my tears would help me because Mamita never left me alone when I cried. And how would she leave me?

However, she turned to me and said, "Everything will be fine, dochenka. I will be waiting for you right here. I'm not going anywhere. I'll be right here until they finish."

"No, I don't want to go, I want to be with you. I don't want to go, Mami, please, I don't want to go with them, I don't want to!" I continued screaming in fear.

The nurses started taking me inside in the bed-car. I squeezed Mamita's hand as hard as I could without letting go. I didn't care how far my arms stretched, but I refused to drop her hand and held on to it for dear life so they wouldn't separate us; but the nurses pushed the wheeled bed hard and managed to tear us apart. They didn't seem to care that I was terrified. I didn't take my eyes off my mommy as they drove me down the aisle, while I kept stretching my arms out, crying and calling out to her. She started to cry too and all I wanted to do was to be with her... I didn't understand why they were taking me away if I didn't want to go.

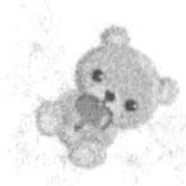 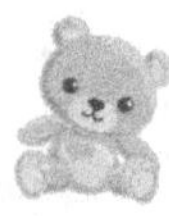 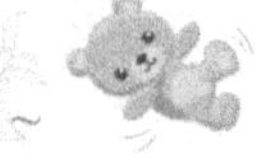 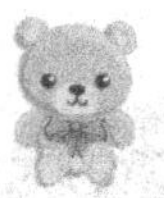

The bed-car kept moving until we stopped ahead in front of a giant door. I was shaking and absolutely terrified! Once the door opened and they got me inside, I could see there were other doctors waiting for me. When the awful people in white passed me through the door, I can't see Mamita anymore and screamed louder, hoping she would come and get me.

Everyone inside the room began to talk to me as the bed-car moved, asking me about my favorite movie or if I liked Mickey Mouse. It sounded like they were trying to calm me down, and I didn't understand know how, but it was working. As soon as one of the doctors saw my nail polish, she looked for a wet cotton ball dipped in a cold liquid to clean it and explained that I couldn't go into surgery with it. I was then pushed into a tiny hallway which was barely wide enough for the bed to squeeze through, and I felt the room shaking. It sounded like I was passing over a bunch of metallic tubes. Finally, I was in a huge room with a number of blinding lamps on the ceiling.

It was so bright and strange there.

"You're cutting my head already? Am I still awake? NO! I don't want that! Please, I don't want that!"

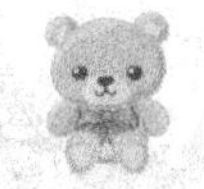 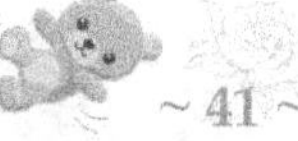 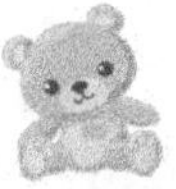 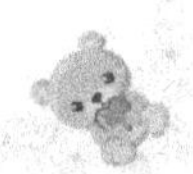

I kept yelling while they were taking me to the operating room. I knew it wasn't hair that they were going to cut that time, but my head. I was extremely worried because I knew how much it hurt when I accidentally cut myself. The doctors tried to calm me down by asking me various questions.

One of them told me, "Look honey, might you hold this for me, please?"

She placed a breathing mask on my mouth and nose. I held it to my face and puff.... I didn't remember a thing after that

EMERGING FROM THE COMA

It felt like another normal Monday and Mamita was waking me up early for school. But something felt strange. I tried to open my eyes, but they didn't respond to me and wouldn't open. I listened to my mommy's sweet voice, and no matter how much I wanted to see her, hug her and never let go of her again, my body wasn't listening to me.

I heard her asking me in the voice I loved, "Do you hear me, dochenka?"

"Yes, Mami! I hear you!" I tried to tell her.

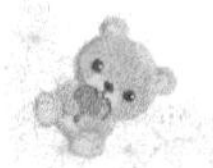
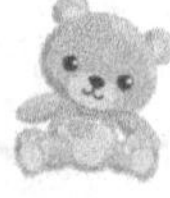
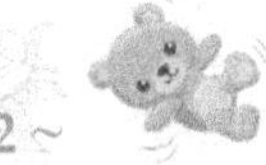
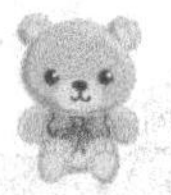

I got no answer – there was only an awkward silence. I didn't understand what was going on! Why couldn't she hear me?

She spoke once more, softly, "Sólnishko moió (my little sunshine, in Russian), Do you hear me?"

"Yes, mommy! I hear you! I hear you! I hear you PERFECTLY!" I repeated several times and made an effort to say it louder to make sure she heard me. Again, nothing.

"What's happening? Mami? Why... why can't you hear me, Mamita? I don't understand anything!"

I wanted to cry. I was answering her questions, but why was she staying silent? Why didn't she hear me? I tried to pronounce the words clearly, but... it was like... somehow... I was trapped in my own body. I couldn't open my eyes either! I didn't know what to do! What was happening to me? What was this? — Then I heard it again.

"Do you hear me... princess, do you hear me? Squeeze my fingers if you hear me, dochenka."

When I heard that, suddenly, I began to feel her fingers in my hand! I felt them! Her warm, soft hand... It was my mommy! What a joy! There she was and I felt her! I squeezed her fingers, but I didn't seem to feel mine. I was not really sure if I was doing it right...

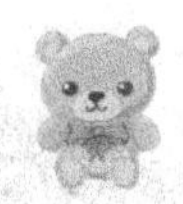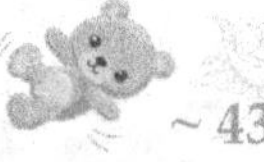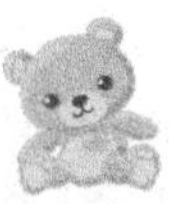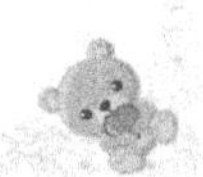

I wanted to do it but my body wasn't responding, or at least, that's what I thought, until Mamita's voice sounded happier than ever when she said, "Yes, you hear me! Thank God you hear me, what a joy! I felt that tiny squeeze, baby!"

I heard her words and it seemed like, yes, I was able to squeeze her fingers!

"Do you understand me, dochenka?" I did it over and over again to reassure her I could hear her.

"You hear me, honey, you understand me!" she goes on, "I'm here, dochenka, I'm right by your side and I'm not leaving you. I'll always stay with you, my little princess. I love you, honey, I love you very much."

I wished that, at that moment, I could hug her and give her a big kiss, but I didn't really understand what was going on. My body didn't do anything I wanted. I couldn't even open my eyes. Did I forget how to do it? It seemed like I was dreaming… but I knew Mamita was real, and that I could feel her hand holding mine. It was a weird feeling. I wanted to wake up.

Later, I heard Babulia's sweet voice ring out, "You are truly strong and brave, Katerina, soon you'll be smiling with us, running all over the place. I love you very much, Katyusha. I admire how brave you are!"

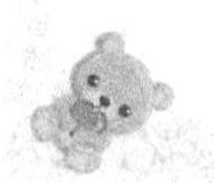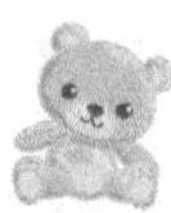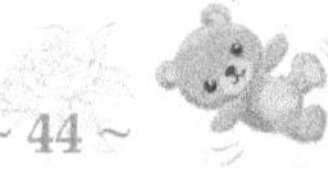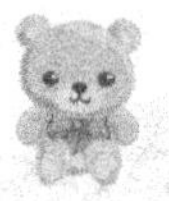

I wanted to give her a big hug too, but I couldn't. She was the best in the world!

A while later, I heard my daddy, "Come on Katerina! You're strong, sweetie. Soon we'll ride the bike together, race and see who wins. We're here with you."

I heard my mommy speaking again.

Was it all happening inside my head? It felt like a dream... even though it seemed so real. I understood everything they were telling me, but I couldn't answer them or move.

"Your brothers Pavel and Klim have arrived. They are by the window, outside the room. If you want me to tell them you said hello, squeeze my fingers." I already knew how to do it, and so I did.

"That's good, princess. I waved to them through the window. They're watching you from outside."

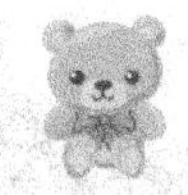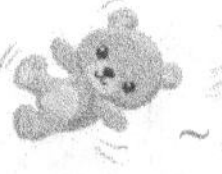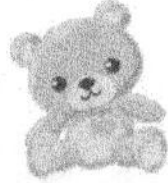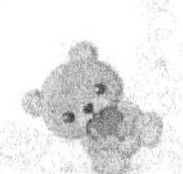

Then, Mamita hugged me and gave me so many kisses, softly whispering to me that Pavel and Klim were happy for my greetings. I wished I could do the same. I thought that the surgery was already over, but I didn't feel anything like my mommy had promised. She seemed to be weeping tears of happiness, it must have been because she knew I was safe; though I couldn't see her, I knew she was by my side.

Step by step, I slowly began to feel my body and realized I could very slightly open my eyes. My head felt heavy. I tried to open my eyes a bit more but the weakness beat me that time; so, I gave up and closed them again. I felt Mamita's arms around me and her voice made me feel instantly better and safer. Was I hugging her back or was my mind playing tricks on me? It seemed I'd fallen asleep soon after because I didn't remember anything.

I panicked when I woke up later because I couldn't see my mommy. My voice had come back so I screamed as loud as I could.

"Where's my mommy? I want to see my mommy! Mami! Mamita! I want to be with Mami! Mami!"

The nurses came running towards me saying, "Calm down Katerina, your mommy is here. Let us call her in for you, don't worry."

I could've filled the room with tears, but my mommy appeared. I could hug her as much as I wanted, finally!

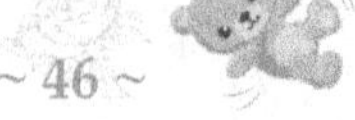
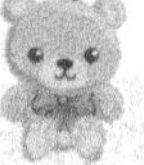

"Mami... Mami, don't go, please don't go! I want to be with you, I don't like it here!" I cried into her arms.

"Yes, baby, yes. I'm here, you finally woke up, princess. I'm not going anywhere. I was waiting for you to wake up, dochenka."

I looked around and saw that it was a big room, with other children sleeping in their beds.

"Where are we, Mami?" I asked her.

"We are in a special room, baby. It's called intensive care. They brought you here after the surgery to take care of you and to make you feel better. How do you feel?"

"My head hurts so much, Mamita. It feels so heavy."

"I know princess, you just had a surgery. It is normal. Try not to move it too much, you have some tubes in there. We hope your head heals fast."

I couldn't move my head. I felt like it was enormous… or like they'd placed a huge rock on top of it. The nurses give me tons of medicine when I couldn't take the pain after a point.

"It hurts so much! It hurts!" The moment she heard my complaints, a nurse ran into the room.

"I'm going to give you morphine to make you feel better."

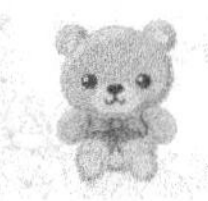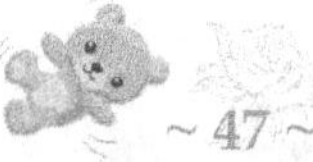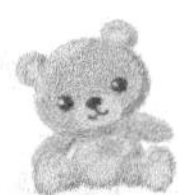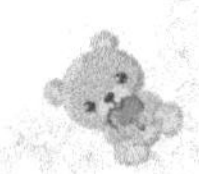

Therefore, every time I was in pain, I know what I had to ask for, so I screamed, "I want morphine, it hurts!" It was indeed a magical medicine because it took away my ache immediately. That was the reason I learned what to ask for since the first time.

I could finally wrap my arms around Mamita. I was so sick of the tubes in my head that wouldn't let me leave the hospital. I desperately wanted to go home with my family. My daddy stayed with me whenever my mommy couldn't. At nights, for example, I was not alone or afraid because watching my daddy next to me whenever I woke up in the dark made me go back to sleep peacefully; poor thing, he took care of me all night without sleep, and it was only when Mamita arrived in the morning that he went home to rest a bit.

My mommy had already arrived and I couldn't stand the position I was in anymore. It was annoying being stuck there and I told her, "I'm very uncomfortable, Mami, always looking at the same side makes me very tired."

"Let's call the nurses, honey, we'll see what they can do," she answered me.

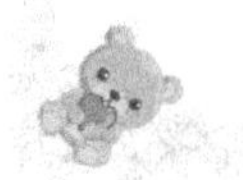
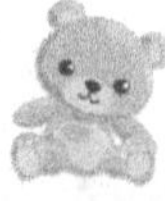

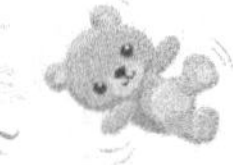
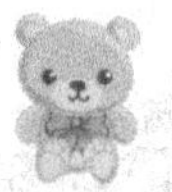

I had a special button to call them, and they came in as soon as I pressed it. Then I explained to them what was bothering me. It didn't really matter how softly or slowly they turned me; my head hurt worse with any movement. And when I was finally made to face the other side, I felt terrible, so I told them, "I don't like it that way, I want to turn back like before!"

The poor nurses turned me back to how I was before. It was a lot of work and they did it lovingly and patiently.

The nurses also bathed me every day. It wasn't how I usually showered, but more like a car wash. They turned me around carefully and used big sponges full of soap to clean my body, then changed all the wet sheets, and, at last, dried me using towels that were as soft as a teddy. I didn't know how, but they did it so well, and those baths always made me feel much infinitely better.

Dr. Poca, the one who had operated on me, visited every day to check up on me, asking me how I was doing, and was always encouraging me; she talked with my mommy about things that I didn't understand at all, but I liked her a lot, even though she always had a serious face.

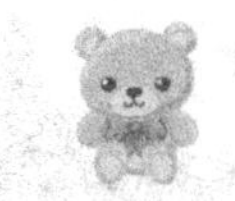 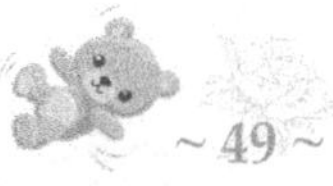 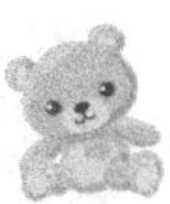 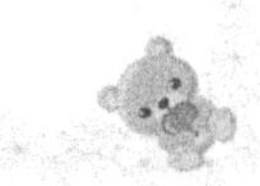

Only one other person was allowed to stay with me in intensive care, so mommy and daddy usually took turns to be with me, unless the hospital staff allowed them in together. Mamita had put up pictures on the wall – there were ones from when I was doing rhythmic gymnastics with my fun tricks (like the split), or family portraits with my cousins and brothers. Oh! They'd made me drawings too and my mommy had found a place to hang them up. They made the place feel more familiar and comfortable for me.

I felt like I hadn't been allowed to eat for years! I could only drink water and was hungry, very hungry! I wanted to at least eat some cookies… or maybe just a snack. I couldn't take it anymore so I called them angrily, "Why don't they give me food? I'm so hungry! I want to eat!

The only thing they brought me was a bowl of broth. A BROTH? I managed to take a few sips but it never made me feel full and I was still hungry once I was done.

A nurse told me, "You can't eat too much at once; it could make you puke and you won't be able to eat again."

I heeded and continued getting tiny sips. I was starving and could have eaten an entire elephant all by myself at that point.

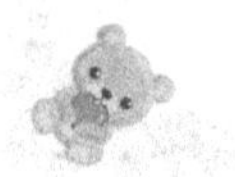 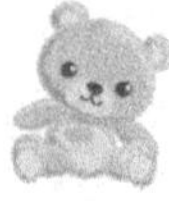 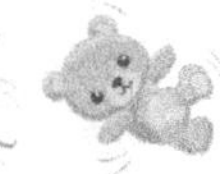 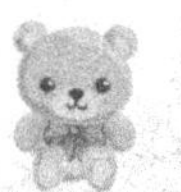

A few days later, Dr. Poca came to visit again and told me, "Are you ready to go to the oncology ward, Katerina?"

"Yes! I'm ready! Are they going to take these things off my head already?"

"Not yet sweetie, but sooner than you think."

"How nice! What a joy!" my mommy exclaimed. "The family can all come and visit you now, baby. And we can all be in the room at the same time, plus we don't have to wear the white coats anymore."

Dr. Poca left the room, and my mommy and I waited for the people that were supposed to transfer me to the oncology ward – the place I'd first arrived at

RECOVERING PROCESS

Two nurses brought the same wheeled bed that had taken me to the surgery room. We were finally out of there!

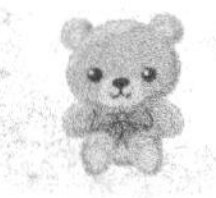
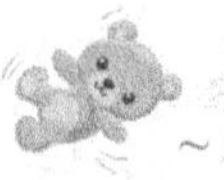
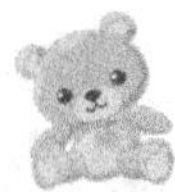
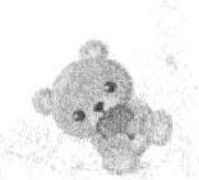

"Oh! Please, don't forget my drawings and my pictures on the wall, Mamita. We can't leave them behind." I was taken to the oncology ward by the nurses who already knew me.

"Welcome Katerina, welcome!" one of them said. "How are you Katerina? How do you feel?" he asked me in a tender voice.

I was finally in a normal room with a big window where you could see the sunlight streaking in. It was daytime. It was a big room with no machines; just my mommy, my daddy and I. There were two beds and no other children were there, except me! My brothers and my family could visit me, and we could all be together! I felt different in that room, as if I were at home.

During the nights, my daddy stayed with me and my mommy went home with my brothers. I didn't want her to leave, but I knew she'd be back early in the morning, once she'd dropped Pavel and Klim off at school. One day, my daddy left the hospital after an argument he had with Mamita. She was very worried about who would stay with me, and called all of her friends, until one of them said he could come and take care of me. One evening, my uncle Ilya kept me company, and my mom came later as usual. So both of them stayed with me overnight. For the next night, a friend of my Mami's watched over me, then another night, someone else, until my daddy came back again.

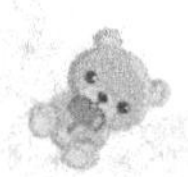 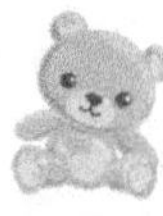 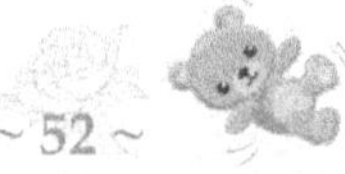 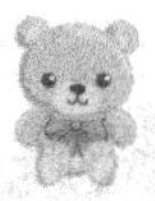

I loved that my mommy brought me different toys to play with. One day, she brought me a new portable DVD with cartoon discs.

Now I could watch my cartoons peacefully since the TV in the room was very old and the pictures could barely be seen. I didn't understand anything they spoke, nor could I hear anything. On the DVD, I had a complete series of Hello Kitty that I could watch non-stop, over and over again. That way, I could spend my days much more entertained since I couldn't get out of bed, or go to the game room with the other kids.

One day, Dr. Poca came in, followed by a few other people, and said they were going to change my bandages. My mommy and daddy were asked to leave the room, and I was so terrified, I started crying. The moment they touched the bandages, I screamed out loud in fear. I felt uncomfortable having them touching my poor little head. It hurt me badly.

HURRAY! I'M STANDING!

One morning, Dr. Poca appeared and told me, "I have some good news, little girl. We're going to take your tubes out today."

"Really?" I ask excitedly.

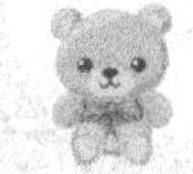
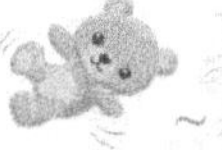
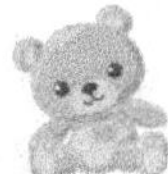
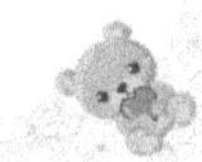

"Yes!" she answered.

They waited for my mommy and daddy to leave to begin the process. I screamed when they took off the bandages and the wires that had stopped me from getting out of bed, for days, but a little bit less than the previous time.

Finally! The bandages were gone. Mamita, yaya, and my uncle Ilya were together that day. They walked into the room once the doctors had finished their work, and jumped for joy when they watched me sitting on the bed for the first time after the surgery.

"Katerina, you're sitting up! And you don't have to be attached to the bed! That poor pillow already has a hole in it!"

We all laughed.

They gave me kisses and congratulated me, because even though my head was still a bit sore and bandaged, there weren't any tubes attached to it. If I wanted to see someone who was out of sight, I had to turn my whole body, along with my head, because I still couldn't move my neck by itself. I felt like a robot, you know?

"I want to stand up. Can I, Mamita?"

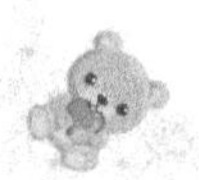
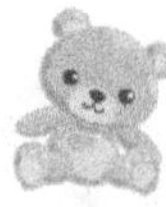
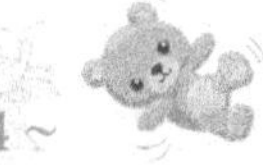
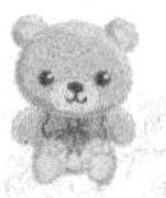

"Sure, honey. Let's try it. The doctors say we can do it carefully, we'll keep an eye on you in case you fall."

Then Mamita and Ilusha helped me stand next to the bed by holding on to me on either side.

"Are you ready, Katerina?" they asked.

"Yes, I'm ready!"

They slowly dropped my hands for a while and YES! I WAS STANDING! I WAS DOING IT ALL BY MYSELF! I felt so happy! Babulia took a picture of me and I smiled for her at the right time. That very moment would be a piece of my story; it was like being born again and learning everything step by step. I could finally go to the bathroom. Ilusha carried me in his arms (he was so strong), and sat me down on the toilet. I didn't want to get up and was happy to do simple activities like that.

"Katerina, what's taking you so long, did you really need to pee?" He wouldn't let me focus, making me laugh so much that I couldn't relax and do my business, which seemed like something I'd never done before in my life.

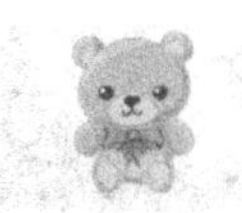
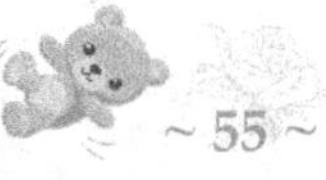
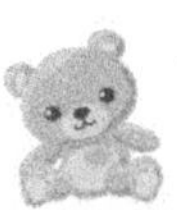
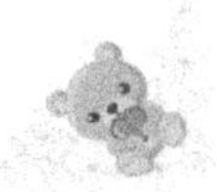

Days went by and I felt stronger. I could sit in a wheelchair and leave the room, and rode all over the place in it. I felt free, even though I wasn't allowed to go outside. I could go to the playroom where I could draw, make necklaces, play legos and board games. The place was always full of volunteers (nice people who liked to help others). Andreu, the famous clown, was there too. He played with me, made lots of jokes and performed magic tricks for us. There were some pictures of us in the hospital magazine, and we quickly became best friends..

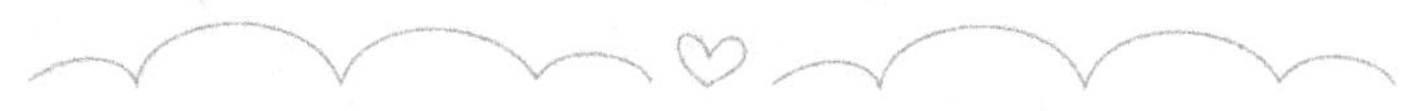

MY BROTHER PAVEL'S BIRTHDAY

My older brother, Pavel's birthday was coming up soon and we were going to celebrate it – not at home, as usual, but at the hospital, because I still wasn't allowed to leave. The whole family was arriving on June 20th and I was going to prepare something special for him.

I was going to give him two gifts; the first one was a very big cardboard boat that I'd been making on my own. I wrapped it in gift paper and put a bow on it. And the second present was a bracelet; it hadn't come out the way I'd expected it to, but my Mamita helped me with it. It was very colorful, and I knew my brother would love it too. Finally, I put the bracelet in a decorated box, wrapped it in gift paper and put a little bow on top as well.

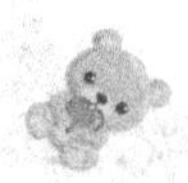
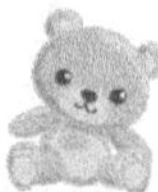
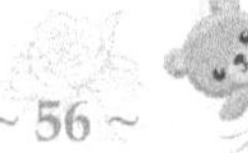
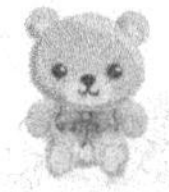

The big day finally arrived! My brother Pavel was turning twelve.

I didn't like the hospital clothes at all. I had to wear the same boy's pajamas every day. It was the only thing I was allowed to wear and they never brought me dresses. However, since it was a special occasion, I was allowed to wear a beautiful dress for Pavel's special day. I liked it very much; it was green with straps that could be tied into little bows on my shoulders. Mamita also tied a white scarf decorated with rhinestones on top of my head's bandages. I was ready! I was so happy when I saw myself in the mirror! I looked beautiful! Everyone arrived one after the other – my aunt Liubasha, my cousins, Melani and Adelina, my granny yaya, my uncle Ilusha, my brothers Pavel and Klim, my mommy and my daddy. So many people! I did indeed have a very big loving family.

Mami bought a big round cake before she came to the hospital. We put candles in the shape of number twelve and sang the birthday song in four different languages as we always did: Russian, Spanish, Catalan and English. Since we sang so much, all the candles had almost burned out. Once we finished, Pavel blew out the candles and we all applauded. Then we could finally got to eat the cake since I loved cakes so much. My favorite flavor was chocolate and Pavel's was lemon... Yummy!

I was the first one to give him the presents!

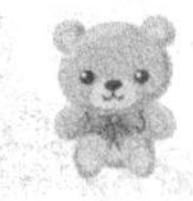
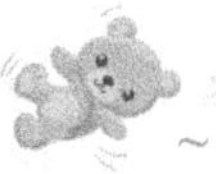
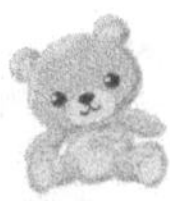
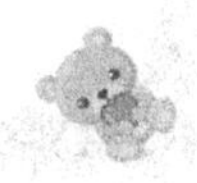

"Happy birthday!" I gave him kisses and hugged him tightly. Smiling, Pavel was excited with his first present.

"Oh, how nice Katerina, you are an artist!" he said lovingly. Then he opened his second present, the one with the bracelet, and got even more excited; probably because of how beautiful it was. We helped Pavel put the bracelet on and it looked so cool on him. He hugged me again and then everyone started giving him their presents too.

In a moment, we started singing again as Liubasha played the guitar my daddy had brought for me (he knew I wanted to learn how to play it), while my family sang funny songs that made us laugh, but then she played a Russian song and they all cried a bit. It had difficult lyrics I didn't really understand, but I knew it was an emotional song… they repeated, several times, something like "I don't want four walls…"

Even though the nurses always gave me medications to soothe the pain, my head still hurt from time to time. Exhaustion took over my body and I didn't have much energy or strength left to stay awake. Thus Mamita laid me down in bed, while Klim took off both my shoes and the scarf, except for the dress. I wanted to sleep in it. Everybody talked so softly, they barely made any noise. I wanted them to stay. It was wonderful to know that we were all together.

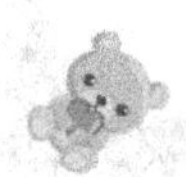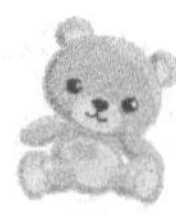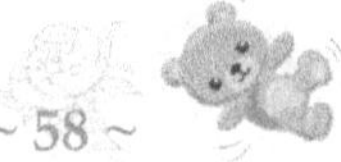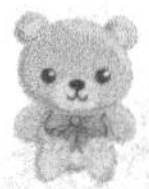

When everyone left, Mamita slid into bed with me. We hugged and she held my hand in hers, while I fell asleep, full of joy and emotion.

MY VISITS

I had another brother whose name was Robin; he was my daddy's son. His girlfriend was really gorgeous, and they'd both come to visit me. They gave me a stuffed mouse: it had a beautiful pink dress… the ears, feet and hands were huge, but the legs and arms were tiny. It was so funny and cute!

Another day, Dr. Pascual, my pediatrician, stopped by. She'd brought me a nice Hello Kitty bag. I liked her very much.

I was also hospitalized the day I was supposed to attend a competition with the girls, and even though, we couldn't dance together, I got two medals and a teddy because my team had won. The trainers came by and gave them to me. They told me that one medal was for winning, and the other one was for having been so brave during the surgery. And finally, the teddy was a present from my classmates. It made me feel so special, as if I had been in the competition performing what we'd learned throughout the year..

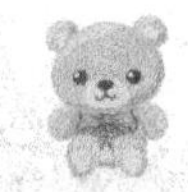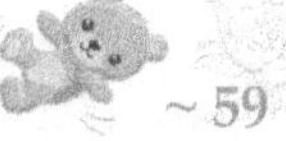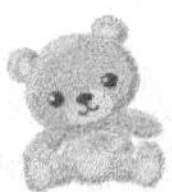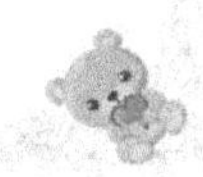

ENOUGH OF HOSPITAL!

The doctors told us we could go home! Hurray! We were finally leaving!

As time went by, Mami had brought me so many things that when we left the hospital, we not only needed lots of suitcases, but also boxes and bags, and it looked like when we were moving houses. I felt free, as if mommy and I were little birds, and someone has forgotten to close our cage. We could finally escape! We were flying away! My daddy drove us in his old car to the house where my brothers and my grandmother were waiting for me.

"Katerina you're here! Finally! We're so happy you're back home, sweetie! Welcome."

I was carefully carried inside and they gave me plenty of kisses. The house smelled great since it seemed babulia had prepared some yummy treats to celebrate my return, and the table had already been decorated for lunch.

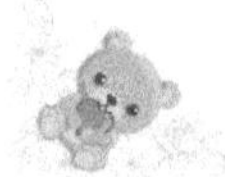
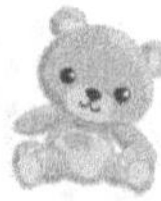
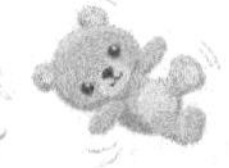
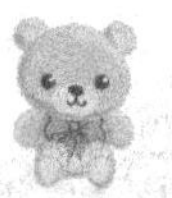

My room remained the same – nothing had changed. My six daughters, and my stuffed animals were happy to see me. I said "hello" and kissed them all, explaining where I'd been, and the reason they hadn't come with me... I'd missed each one quite a bit. They also met their four new sisters: a little mouse, a white bear and two more Hello Kitties (a big one dressed in pink with a pearl necklace, and a smaller one). Our family was bigger now.

I was changing my babies' dirty clothes and giving them food, while Mami helped babulia set the final touches for the welcome party. The girls were very supportive and none of them were angry at me; just a bit sad. They were good daughters, as I was with Mami. They listened to what I told them and it made me happy they were that educated. It was probably how Mamita felt when I listened to her.

Since it was lunchtime, my mommy helped me sit at the table and brought me my plate. We always started the meal with a green salad that had lettuce, tomatoes, onion, cucumber, and other vegetables whose names I couldn't recall; once we'd finished, it was time for the second dish: chicken with mashed potatoes, and we had some iced tea as well. I was drooling. It was my first meal after returning home... how different it felt.

It was good to be there.

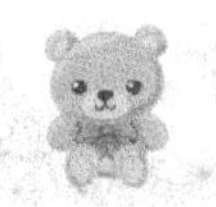
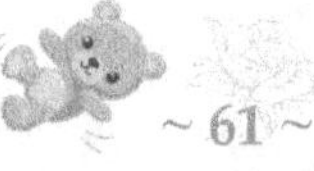
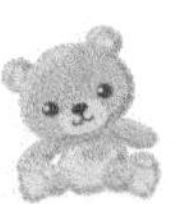
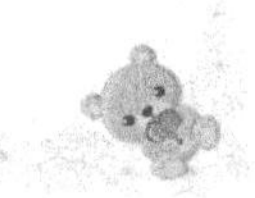

No doctor was going to check up on me a thousand times a day, nor would anyone wake me up early. There were no sick people around, or scary machines. I also didn't have to stay in bed all day, but you know the best part? My mommy's amazing food! And being able to spend time with my brothers without having to say goodbye. Besides, sleeping in those boring sheets at the hospital was a real nightmare – my room was much cozier, with my favorite toys, my dolls and the princess's blankets.

Our house was fantastic! A dream kitchen, a Japanese style living room, colored with red, black and white, with swings and ropes hanging from the middle of the ceiling, so we could do some stunts. I knew I couldn't do them yet, but I could play with my daughters there, right?

In two days, Pavel and Klim would be going to the camp they went to every summer vacation to learn English. I couldn't go yet because I wasn't old enough. But I didn't want to either, since I'd rather stay with my mommy. The place was a bit far from home, so a friend of Mami's offered to go with us. I got into the front seat of the car, leaning it back so my head could rest. It was weird that holding it up was still difficult; and so was standing or walking. I got tired quickly, and when that happened, my mommy's friend carried me in his arms since he was super strong. We dropped my brothers off at the summer camp and went for a walk in the park straightaway, hoping to find some nice restaurant.

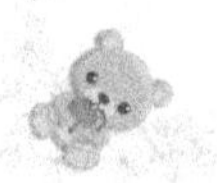 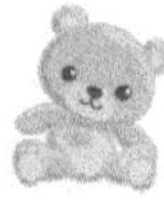 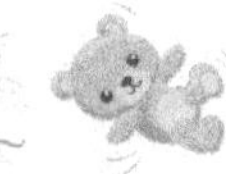 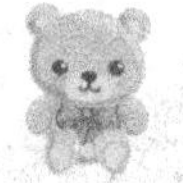

NO MORE BANDAGES

Soon the patches that wouldn't let me move my head would be gone. We arrived at the doctor's office, where she asked me to sit down next to the table and rest my head on my arms.

"I'm scared, Mami," I said, looking at her.

"It won't hurt, baby. It's like a mosquito bite, you'll see," the doctor answered and I listened to her, but I was still frightened. "You have 28 staples, Katerina, and today we're going to take out only 14…which is half of them."

I was even more scared on hearing her! 28? And she was going to take out only half of them? The nurse rubbed my head with something wet and then started to take the staples off, one by one. I was sweating and squeezing mommy's hand.

"Oh no! It hurts!"

"Hang in there, Katerina," the nurse encouraged, so I held on as long as I could. "There, Katerina, we're done. Let me just put a new patch on you and that's it, you're ready."

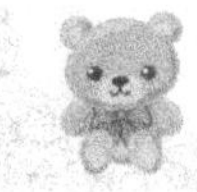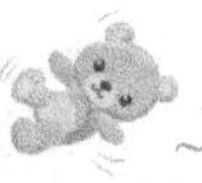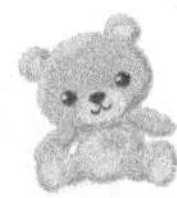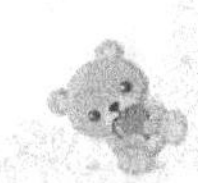

'Ugh! That was scary,' I thought to myself.

The moment we left the doctor's office, Mamita told me, "You see how fast that was? Did it hurt?"

"It didn't hurt too much, Mami, but it was scary. I can move my head a little better now."

"That's great, honey."

"Yes, I feel much better... I wonder when they're going to take the rest off."

"We have to be patient. Soon you won't even have one single staple."

My mommy was right! We would be going back to have the rest of the 14 staples removed. Then, I would be able to move my head even better. It would be amazing!

I still wore scarves on my head because I didn't have any hair yet, although, it was starting to grow a bit and forming spikes. I was like a hedgehog. I wasn't worried because it was still summer, and mommy told me that by the time we started school again, my hair would be a bit longer. In the meantime, we were going to the doctor again to continue my astronaut modeling session (I finally knew it was called an MRI).

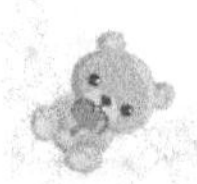 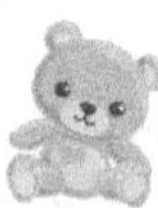 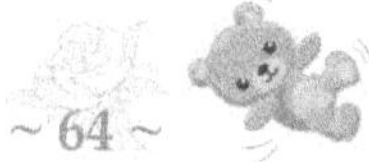 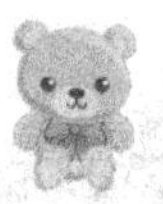

I got a brand-new princess bike – it was pink and lilac, like my room. It had two big wheels and two small ones at the back; I liked riding it, except when there was a steep climb. Then it was very hard for me. It was a good thing my mommy helped me and pushed from behind. Being on vacation was the best! One day, we went out to the park and saw David, a classmate; I think he was curious about the hat I was wearing because it completely covered my head. So, he came over and tried to pull it off of my head, but, thank God, my mommy was there! She stopped him right away and told him he shouldn't do that. David ran away, scared. What a bully!

By the way! My brothers came back from the summer camp, and finally we were all together, playing tricks on each other.

We went back to the hospital to see the oncologists. During the summer, we'd visited the doctors so many times that I'd already memorized their names. There were three of them: Dr. Gallego, whom I liked a lot because she was very gentle and loving with me, Dr. Sábado, whom we joked around with and called Domingo (which meant Sunday in spanish, while his name meant Saturday), and Dr. Díaz, who was a super serious man with a very deep voice. Dr. Sábado enjoyed having really long conversations with my daddy.

When we went into the office to talk to Dr. Gallego, she said, "It's time to start chemotherapy."

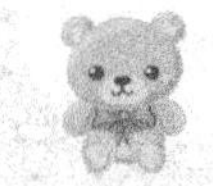
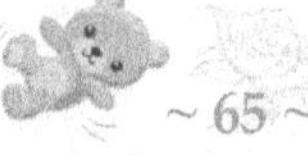
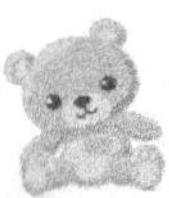
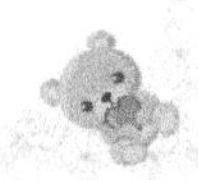

They talked about my new treatment, but I didn't understand anything, nor did I know what it meant... it sounded kind of scientific. They gave us a long list of dates and another round of medicines that I had to take. They also mentioned that I had to go back to the operating room again, to put on, I didn't know what.

"What is it?" I asked. "I don't want to go there, ever again!" I said, scared. I hadn't liked that place the last time.

"We need to insert a small piece under your collarbone." I didn't even know what a collarbone was, much less where it was.

"It's about the size of a coin but elastic, like silicone, and it'll help make your treatments easier. It'll be quick, it doesn't hurt, and you won't feel a thing."

"I don't want to have another surgery!"

"It won't hurt, honey. Plus, you'll be asleep like last time and it'll be much, much faster. It's just a very small cut." I didn't like the idea at all.

When I got home, I asked my mommy, "What's chemo... Mamita?"

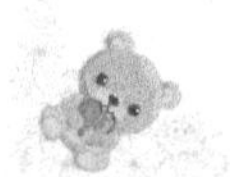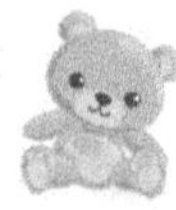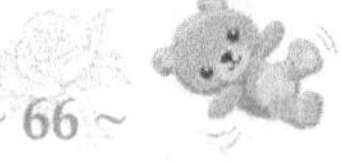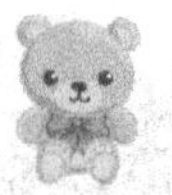

"It's a special treatment, princess. They put you on liquid medicine for a couple of hours. We're going to do this new treatment at the hospital for a few months... a couple of hours once a week. Don't worry, we won't sleep there. This treatment is special, baby girl, you might lose some hair... But that doesn't always happen."

"What hair, Mami? My hair is barely growing and it is already really short."

"I know honey, but never mind, maybe we're lucky and that won't happen, but if it does, I'm sure it will grow back again, prettier and stronger."

"Why do they want to give me that treatment, Mami?"

"Well...The doctors want to make sure the nut doesn't grow back. Remember? They only removed a bit, and we don't want it to bother you again, right?"

"No, I don't want it to grow, and I don't want it to be in my head either."

My mommy then stuck a new colorful and prettier board on the fridge that contained all the instructions the doctors had given us. She'd written down each important date on it and it was huge. She told me the schedule covered a span of two years.

"Wow! That much, Mami? I'm going to be eight years old then!"

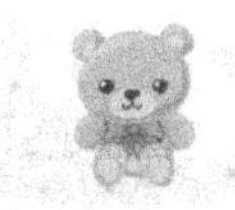
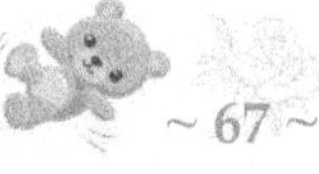
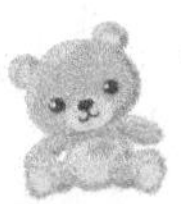
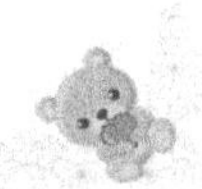

"Yes, sweetie, that's right. But remember, we're not doing it every day so time will go by quickly."

She explained what each square on the board meant, and the exact days that we had to go to the hospital. It was a good thing I didn't have to stay at the hospital, and instead, had to visit every once in a while; for example, we had to visit every Thursday. We bought the medicines I needed to take and wrote them down on the chart too. I even knew all their names and what they were for!

"Here, dochenka, we are going to mark the sessions that have been done so we can know clearly how many are left." It was getting too much! That coin under my collarbone, the "chemotherapy" thing, all those medicines, and the hospital... dear God! I didn't want it!

And just like that, our visits to that creepy hospital began again. The doctors were going to put the coin they'd talked about on our last visit, the "Port-a-Cath" or something like that. We were in oncology already, where I'd had the surgery, and walking through those halls gave me goosebumps. I didn't like it one single bit.

I fell asleep and felt nothing, so it looked like they'd kept their promise after all.

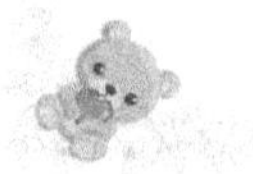 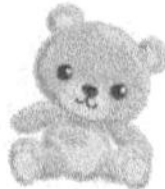 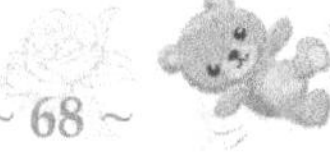 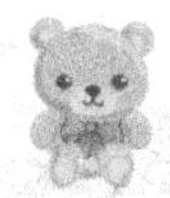

When I woke up, I felt kind of sore. I noticed a round thing under my chest's skin. It looked like a tiny lump, as if I had hit the wall. Ugh… It couldn't possibly be true that the coin was going to be there for the next three years... I wanted the doctors to take it out of me immediately!.

CHEMOTHERAPY

I started my really intense days of treatment ten days before the first day of school. When we arrived at the hospital, the first thing they did was take my blood while I was in the playroom. There were many children there, some crying out loud and being afraid of needles, poor things. I didn't cry since the injections were actually quick and continued playing afterwards. In the meantime, we were to wait for the blood tests' results.

In the "Day Hospital" area where the chemotherapy was done, there were a number of children, but they were really quiet. Some were sitting on their beds with IVs attached, or were sleeping, while others were even watching cartoons; these children weren't crying so I guessed the treatment wasn't painful, thank God! I was supposed to start the sessions soon and mommy told me it would last a few hours, even though we were not going to be staying the night. Someone brought me food, like I was getting admitted. It was nice to play or draw while the treatment was in progress through my collarbone coin.

One Thursday, we were already at the hospital and were waiting for the usual test results when the doctor called us inside his office. He told us that they wouldn't be giving me any treatment because my blood needed to heal, or something like that. Some other Thursday, I was so weak that I got something called a "blood transfusion", and it seemed I was missing another thing called "platelets". Anyways, the whole ordeal took my strength away. Indeed, I'd learned lots of new words, hadn't I? The sad thing was that the dates had changed, which meant my mommy had to make a new board.

THE SCHOOL

Three hard months had passed since the surgery and we were all ready to go back to school, again. Remember the building that I'd told you about? The big one where Pavel and Klim were studying? It was my first day there! It felt great! When we arrived, I lined up, as usual, and waited for the other children and for the teacher to pick us up. My classmates looked at me curiously, and I started feeling uncomfortable.

"Katerina, Katerina, what's wrong with you? Why are you wearing a headscarf?" they asked me.

"Well, because I like it."

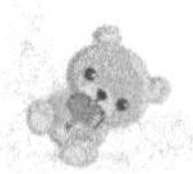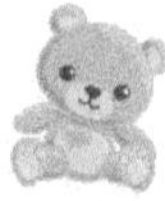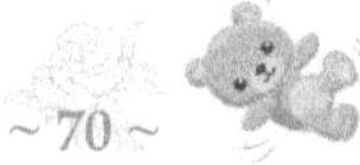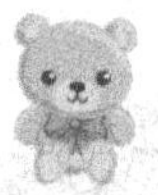

They gave me another odd look, trying to understand my answer, or so I thought. It was better they didn't know what was going on, just so they wouldn't bother me with dumb questions. My secret was safe and nobody was going to get it out of me, no matter what happened. I didn't have any trouble keeping secrets because I did it quite often with my brothers and Mamita.

"Dochenka, how do you do it?" Mami would always ask me, surprised.

To be honest, it felt like a game to me. I felt super important and responsible and knew I couldn't tell anyone. That was how it was done.

Did I tell you Mami was my best friend? We even had sleepovers once every three days; I mean, my brothers did it too, so I had to wait for my turn to sleep in her giant bed. Unless she wanted to sleep alone, then I had to wait extra days. But I didn't care much because Pavel and Klim sometimes forgot about it and I got to stay many more nights with her; it was so difficult to give up any sleepover time with Mami, but I had to do it whenever my brothers remembered the deal. They just didn't understand I didn't want to leave her, ever!

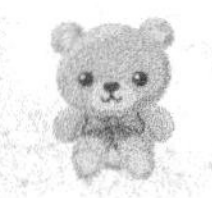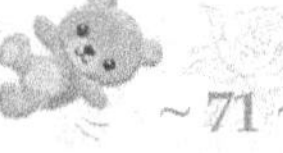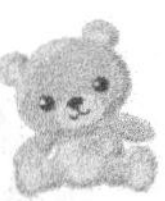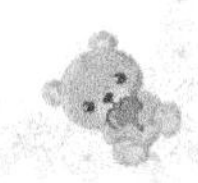

I loved going places with my mommy, and she always held my hand. I held on to tight so I wouldn't lose her, and if she did let go, I quickly held on to her skirt until I saw her hand get free again. I was clingy, and without Mamita's hand or skirt, panic overcame me.

CHEMOTHERAPY CONTINUES

I'd learned our routine pretty well by that point: once a week, we had to go to the hospital, I would get the analysis, wait in the playroom for the doctors to call us in, go to the special room where I had to undergo the chemo for a few hours, and finally, we went home. It was always the same. Like clockwork. The best thing about the treatment was that I ended up getting so tired that I didn't have to go to school. There were days when I didn't feel as bad and I could play with my siblings. On some days, I felt awful and I stayed in bed all day with a tummy ache. And so, the weeks dragged on.

My mommy explained the two main treatments to me: one with Vincristine, which was short, just one injection and we were home (I even went back to school sometimes), and the other one with Carboplatin, which was endless. Each treatment made me feel different – some made me feel better, while others drained my energy and I wanted to throw up.

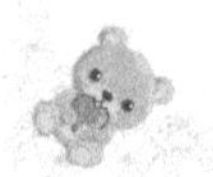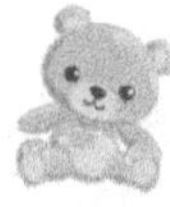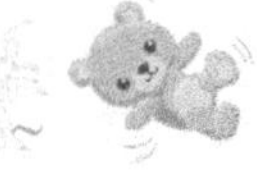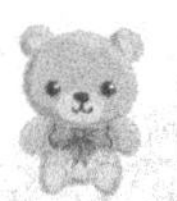

Something I didn't like about the chemotherapy was that, somehow, the food didn't taste the same. I didn't even like my favorite food anymore, not even chocolate covered donuts. I was completely disgusted by them, and plus, if I ate more than just a little bit, I went into a food coma. So I wasn't hungry most of the time.

I still had to take tons of medications every day and it was a never-ending story. Sometimes, the heartburn or headaches were terrible and I completely lost my appetite. Whenever that happened, I avoided staying alone in my room and my mommy would rest on the living room couch with me. She put some blue jelly-like thing in a bag which made me feel better, and it had a warm or cold texture.

The few hairs I had fell out almost entirely. Nevertheless, when I turned seven, the sessions were spaced further apart from each other, and my hair started growing back slowly. At one point, I finally had enough hair for a boy's cut and I could go to school without a headscarf. My classmates still made fun of me but I ignored them because I knew they were children (almost babies), and they didn't really understand what was going on. My mommy told me that the time lapse between the sessions was a blessing and allowed me to recover, which was why my hair wasn't falling out anymore. Soon I'd be like Princess Rapunzel!

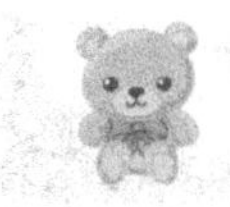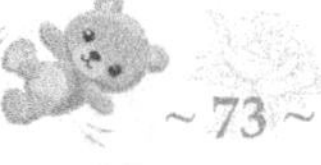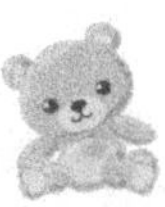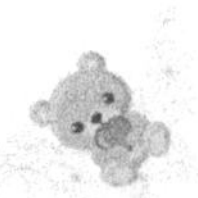

We'd finally reached the final goal of chemotherapy! The last day was on March 30th, 2011, and I was excited! It meant that 88 weeks had passed since the beginning of the treatment.

On the day of my last chemo, the oncologists told us that we had to repeat the MRI the following month, and if everything went right, we only had to return every five or six months for a check-up; time passed quickly and the doctors had begun making several imaging tests, checked my tumor's behavior and found it'd gotten smaller... which meant no more treatment!

We were free from the hospital! My hair had grown back completely and I looked like a girl again!

SURPRISE TRIP!

I turned eight and grew even bigger and smarter. I was almost done with the second grade; Klim was at the end of the sixth, so he was going to start high school the following year and would be leaving me alone in primary. It had been awesome having my brother by my side and defending me from the bullies out there. I knew I had to do it by myself.

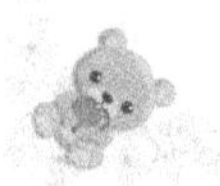
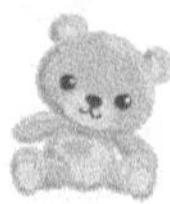
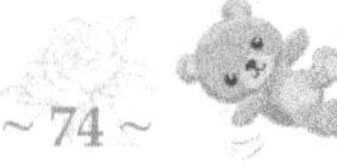
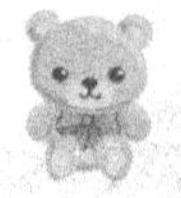

Pavel was no longer in the same school as us since he was finishing his second year in a high school on the other side of the road. Since his schedule was different from ours, he'd leave home earlier. For the remaining months, Klim and I went to school alone. Just the two of us.

May came around quickly! Three gloriously peaceful months passed without a treatment session, and the end of the school year was around the corner. It was a quiet Friday evening at home! Mamita, Pavel and I enjoyed some time together at home, while Klim was at his best friend, Albert's house.

Someone knocked at the door and we raced to see who would open it first (it was our favorite game). My mommy won that time. Klim, Albert, his little sister and his dad were standing at the entrance. Once they greeted each other, Mami and Albert's dad started talking about the place Klim would be going to study at afterwards. We were all listening carefully because none of us knew about it.

"We're going to another country, Ireland, to be precise." Well, that was a surprise.

"What? Ireland?" Klim interrupted, but Mamita kept talking to the man.

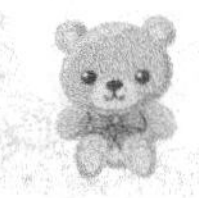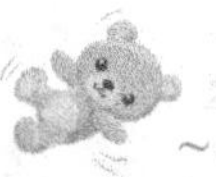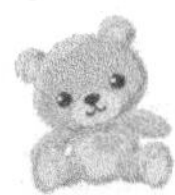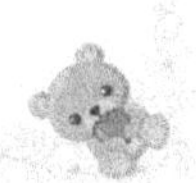

"I haven't talked to my children about this yet, as you see." She turned to us. "I'll explain later." Then went back to the conversation while we listened even more closely. We still couldn't understand anything though.

"I want my children to study for, at least, a year in another country where they speak English, you know… to improve their language skills." Albert's dad was surprised. And we are twice that, but also excited to hear about the plan. The moment our visitors left, we attacked mom with questions.

"Tell us! Tell us mommy! Where are we going?"

"How do you feel about going on a big ship like the Titanic, across the Atlantic Ocean, then driving all over France and Ireland? I'm sure living in Ireland will be an adventure."

"What are you talking about, Mami?"

"I want you to learn the best possible English. It's a very important language worldwide that will open many doors for your future." We paid keen attention to what she said.

"Then we'll come back to Spain. What do you guys think?"

We were all happy and excited because a new experience awaited us. It would be fun to live in another country and speak another language.

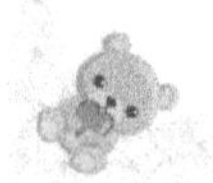
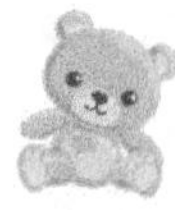
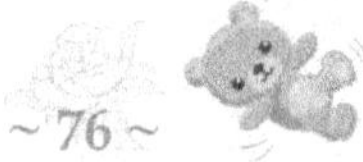
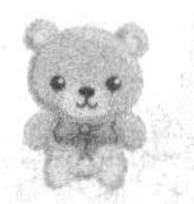

Mamita showed us a few houses she'd looked up on the internet, and we were supposed to choose the one we liked the best to live in. So fun! All of them were huge. She talked to us about the journey and showed us where Ireland was on the map. She pointed out the route we'd follow... I didn't really understand most of it, but it sounded like a movie story and everyone was excited.

"We need to save some money for the trip. I thought we could go to a friend's house in Tarragona, for about three months, so I don't have to pay rent."

I thought it sounded like a nice idea because mommy's friend lived near babulia, and I would be able to see her whenever I want. Besides, my daddy lived there too – we would be able to make his famous big rectangular pizzas together.

"We are going to drive there, and we won't be able to take much with us, only the most important things. I planned the trip for August."

She showed us the map once again, explaining in detail.

"First, we get to the French coast to board a big boat with the car, and then we cross the Atlantic Ocean to Ireland."

"Sounds great!" I shouted.

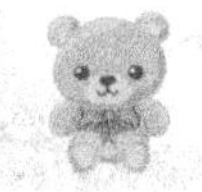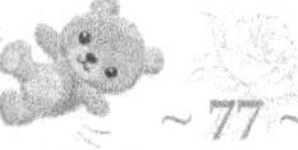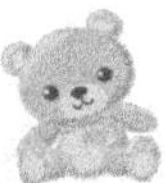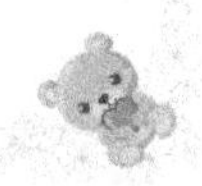

"When we get to Ireland, the most beautiful house you've chosen will be ours. Once we settle in, the only thing left to do is to find a new school, the nearest one. You're going to meet new kids, and have new friends! It's fantastic, isn't it?"

"All right, all right, we want to go!" Pavel and Klim answered, screaming with joy, and I joined them.

"Yes! We want to! New friends sound great!" I didn't really have many.

The previous year, I'd met my brothers' father, Anatoliy, who'd come from Russia to spend time with them. He was supposed to arrive soon, but mommy had already made the plan, so he had to wait for our return the following year. It was sad because he was a good person who loved us very much.

In the meantime, Anatoliy had moved into Klim's room and my mommy was helping him settle down in Barcelona and find a job. He didn't speak Spanish. Sometimes the poor man would ask me what a word meant and I'd help him learn like I was his teacher!

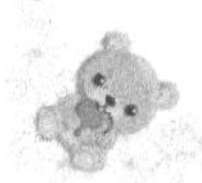
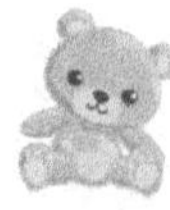
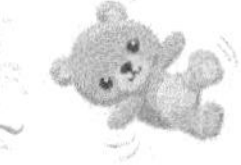
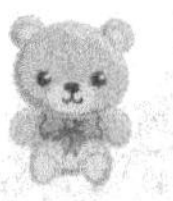

In May, we all moved to Andrés' house in Tarragona…well, except for Klim. He'd decided to stay in Barcelona with Liubasha, but came to visit us on weekends. That day, we'd carried so many things I wondered how they were going to fit in mommy's friend's place, for god's sake! All this house moving almost made me forget mommy was the smartest lady in the universe, and that she would get by.

Klim didn't want to leave school until he finished elementary. The water polo and swimming team trained hard every afternoon in preparation for a competition at the end of the year, so my brother was really busy. I worried constantly because I didn't understand how he could live alone by himself.

I was, however, excited to start the new school in Tarragona, and so was Pavel, even if it was just for a few months. The truth was we had no friends at our old one; Besides, my big brother was rebellious and wanted to get away from his school in Barcelona because it was too strict and religious. Mommy got called to the Principal's office sometimes, and both of them came back home crying. It must have been a big deal seeing how they were both in that state.

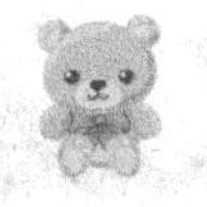 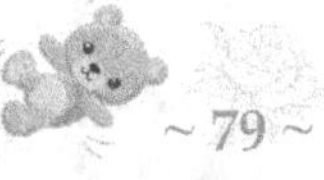 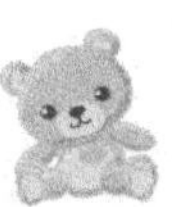 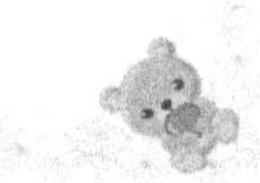

The new environment proved to be a wonderful opportunity for Pavel who was finishing his freshman year in Tarragona because everybody loved him. We were bursting with happiness. Meanwhile, Klim was still struggling to finish elementary school and his competitions, no matter what it took. I admired how brave he was despite being just 12 years old! How did he manage without Mami? He wasn't much older than us. There was no way I could do that! I would have probably lose my mind first!

Once we finished the school year, we enjoyed the summer in Tarragona, going to the beach, meeting new friends, celebrating birthdays, or visiting babulia and my daddy very often, all together again. Plus, the trip to Ireland proceeded smoothly while we ironed out the final details. The online English course was truly fun, and every day I connected with people from many different countries while we learned as a team. The teachers gave us tons of exercises and we improved quickly. My brothers were on a higher level because they knew more than I did. They were lucky to be old enough to go to the summer camp I'd talked about, but I had to start from scratch. We didn't buy anything in Spain so we wouldn't have to carry a lot of things. My mommy said we could buy everything we needed in Ireland.

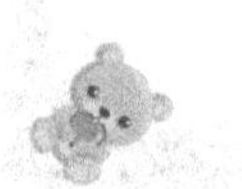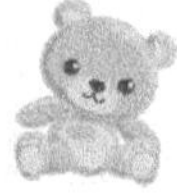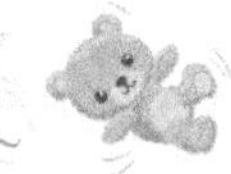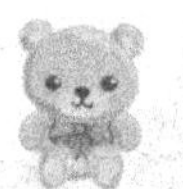

I loved the summers because most of my family's birthdays fell in that season – my uncle Ilusha's on June 5th, fifteen days later was Pavel's on June 20th, then July with Adelina's on the 8th, my mommy's and my aunt Liubasha on the 9th of August , and my granny yaya's on August 12th. My birthday falls on September 28th, so it doesn't fall in Summer, but I still have a good time with them.

My daddy checked mommy's car before we left, so it wouldn't break down during the trip leaving us stranded and not knowing what to do. Just to be sure. She had an old, small car, but it worked just fine.

MAKE A WISH

Mommy told us that we'd gotten a call from a company that made special children's dreams come true, and it was called "Make a Wish".

"We were lucky that Katerina was selected. Sweetheart, you need to choose the most challenging of your dreams, the one that seems almost impossible to realize."

"Me? WOW! Making my dreams come true… but Mami, do you know how many dreams I have? How will I choose one?"

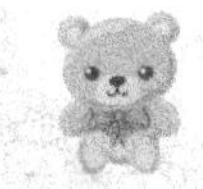
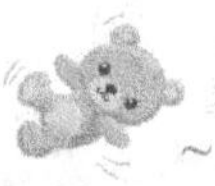
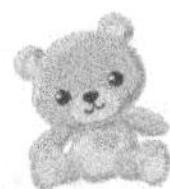
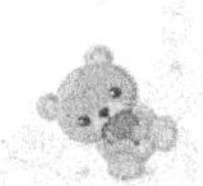

"We'll let's figure it out, baby. The other children have lots of wishes too, but the company helps realize only the biggest one. I'm sure that dream is on the tip of your tongue, honey," she explained. "See, there's this boy that wanted to fly in a helicopter, another wanted to have dinner with Leo Messi, who is a famous soccer player... oh, and there's this kid who wanted to meet his father, "Make a Wish" also took a child to Disneyland, could be Paris or Orlando."

"How's the Park in Orlando like, Mamita? Where is it?"

"Oops! That one is far, far away. It's in the United States, on another continent and another part of the planet. Actually, there are many parks, like Princesses palaces, the Harry Potter themed park, and several more characters... but it is far away and not so easy to get there."

"Do Rapunzel and Tiana live there?"

"Yes, honey, of course. They have their castles there."

"Then I want to go. We've been to the Paris' park, and they didn't have castles. I want to go to the biggest one." I made my decision quickly. Without having second thoughts.

Our entire family attended the interview, Mamita, my brothers and I. When we got there, a lady named Lourdes who was the organizer, welcomed us.

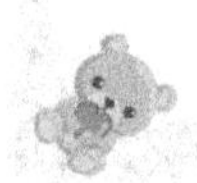 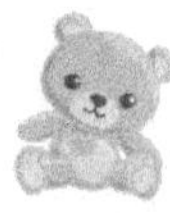 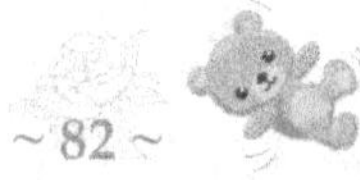 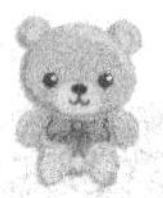

"Nice to meet you, Katerina. Do you know we selected you to achieve your most desired wish?" she asked me. "Tell me what you want to do, baby girl."

"My dream is to meet Princess Rapunzel and Princess Tiana at Disneyland Park in Orlando."

"Well… that park is very far from here, but we can arrange the same in Paris. It will have the same characters, attractions, and much, much more."

I wanted to go to where Rapunzel and Tiana lived. How was it possible for them to be in two places at the same time? Ugh. I didn't understand a thing, but they kept talking so, so much, that at the end I got confused and said, "Okay then, let's go to Paris."

"Great! Your brothers and your mommy can go with you. They'll be your guests."

"All together?"

"Naturally."

"That's great!"

"Before you get your wish, you have to do some homework, right?"

"Sure!" I said, before leaving Lourdes' office and returning home.

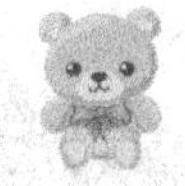 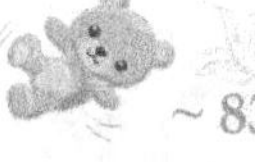 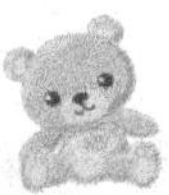 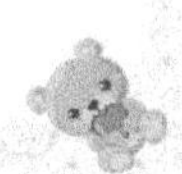

We were supposed to draw my favorite princesses on a huge piece of paper. We were pretty good at it. Pavel was drawing Tiana and Klim is drew Rapunzel, while I colored their dresses by putting glitter everywhere. Oh my God, the entire house was sparkling by the time we were done. We also wrote letters for the pilots. Once we finished, everything was delivered to Lourdes' office, and they really loved it.

On the way home, my brothers asked me, "Katerina, why didn't you keep the wish? I mean, to go to the park in Orlando. We could never go there because it is too far and it costs too much money. Paris is next door."

I thought about it for a moment and then decided I didn't want to go anywhere. They were right. Paris was exciting, but not as much as Orlando. We would literally cross the planet to see all those magical characters, all of them! So, I told mommy that I'd be wasting the opportunity to fulfil my dream.

"In Paris, it's nice too, sweetie, there are lots of different characters and attractions." she told me.

"Yeah, Mamita, but I already know how it is. Moreover, we're going to Ireland soon and I'd rather not go."

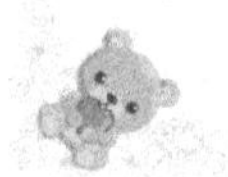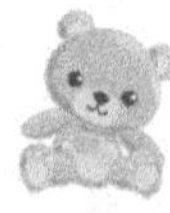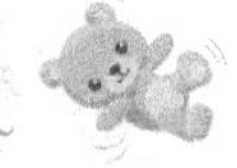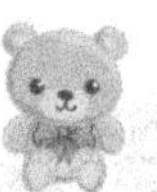

At that moment, my mommy called the company, apologizing for the inconvenience and letting them know our decision. That was it, my dream ended where it began.

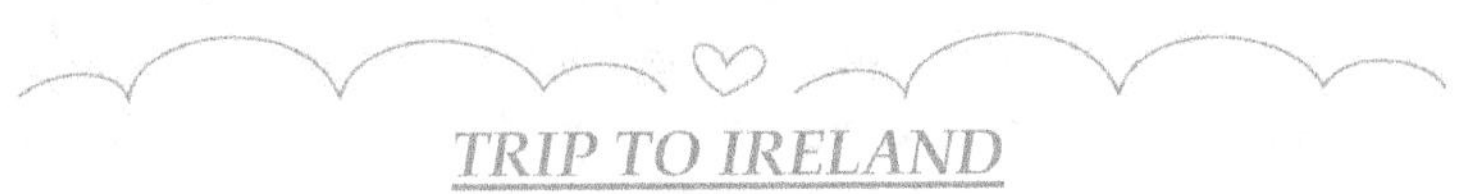

TRIP TO IRELAND

On the morning of August 8th, 2011, as soon as summer ended, we stuffed all our bags and luggage for the Ireland journey into the car, which despite being really small, was able to fit quite a lot of luggage. Klim and I sat in the back seat, separated by a pile of bags placed between us, right up to the car's ceiling. I could barely see him. There were stuff everywhere! Under our feet, the front seat – in fact, the whole car was packed, except mommy's space since she was the driver. We even had a box with snacks for the road trip.

Babulia, daddy, Anatoliy and Andrés helped us pack everything, and when we all took our places, ready to go, everybody came by to say goodbye. We waved our hands out the windows, smiling at them. Our exciting journey to Ireland had begun and I had a feeling that we were entering a fairy tale.

We'd brought some films to watch on the portable DVD player along the way, but it constantly stopped in the middle and turned out to be useless. We were looking for alternatives to entertain ourselves when Mamita said, "In a few minutes we're going to cross the border, guys! We're almost in France."

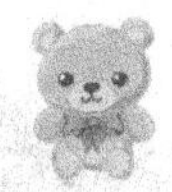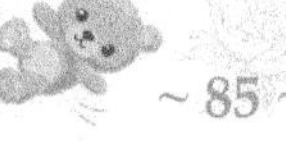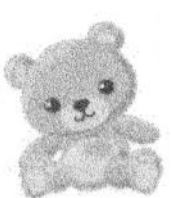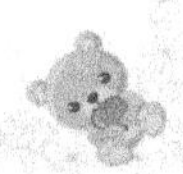

'Wow! Spain and France are really close…' I thought to myself.

It turned out I was learning some geography on the way, and it was way more interesting than on paper or a map. It was an education I'd never forget.

We arrived at a rest area next to a river for our first stop in France. There were many trees around, along with a few wooden tables and stools. I saw many other tourists enjoying their break, so Mami took out our portable fridge with yummy food, and let us play for a little while, running all over the place. The river was not too deep, as my brothers found out by wandering into the water. It only covered their feet; nevertheless, while Pavel was playing, his flip-flop slid off and the waves took it away so fast he didn't have enough time to catch it. Mamita got a bit cross with him after we couldn't find it and said we had to look for a shop to buy new ones.

We continued our journey for about four more hours, making several stops on the way, whether it was to buy some food or because I had to pee, and of course, when the gasoline ran out, mommy stopped at the gas stations. On the way, we listened to rap music by "Nastya & Potap", Russian singers whom Pavel enjoyed listening to. He'd brought an album we'd heard a thousand times before, so much so that we already knew each song by heart.

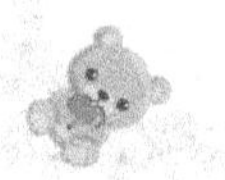
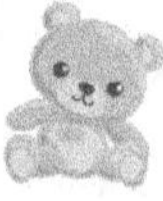
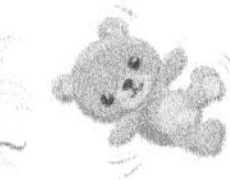
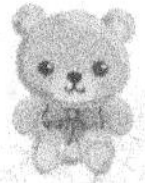

As soon as it started getting dark, Mami started looking for someplace to spend the night. We arrived at a Hotel called "Formula One" in the Niort city, France. The room we got had a bunk bed, so my brothers and I got to sleep on the bottom, which was a double bed, while Mamita took the top, single bed. We took turns to shower before going to rest, and to my horror I realized we'd left all of my panties in Spain. I couldn't believe I'd forgotten them. In any case, mommy assured me she'd buy me some nice, tight ones, but she told me we couldn't make any more stops, so I had to make do with the small panties.

Mommy spent another whole day driving. We stopped at one more hotel in Nantes city where we were able to rest much better. Plus, she told us we could definitely sleep in since we didn't have to wake up early the following day.

On the third day of the trip, we visited Brest city, and mommy drove less and stopped sooner at our next rest stop. The place where we stayed that third time was so much bigger and comfortable, and our room even had four beds, one for each.

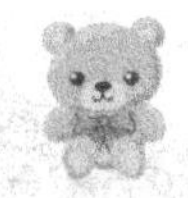
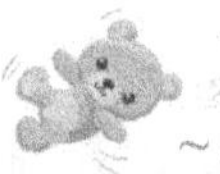
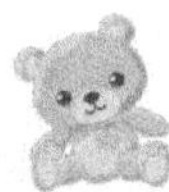
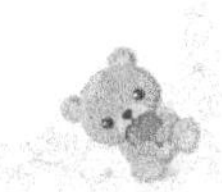

There was no rush. We had enough time in the afternoon to visit the park and goof around after sitting in the car for so long. Mamita told us that we were about an hour away from Roscoff, the upcoming city. To be honest, there was nothing special about it. The spoken language sound similar to Catalan, but a bit weird…To me, it felt like I could understand it, and at the same time, I didn't.

WE'RE CROSSING THE OCEAN!

The trip to the port after leaving the hotel flew by quickly. Roscoff was huge and the ships were as big as the Titanic. We arrived very early and there was still plenty of time to get on board. In the meanwhile, we went for a walk around the city, browsed through a number of shops and bought some food. We'd travelling by boat! My brothers and I kept repeating "How much longer? How much longer?" to mommy the entire time because we were really excited about the adventure that awaited us.

The hours seemed to go on forever, but the time had come. Finally! There were two long lines of cars at the harbor, waiting to get on board.

"I don't understand how all of these cars will fit there… how will the boat hold up? Isn't it going to sink, Mamita?" we asked her.

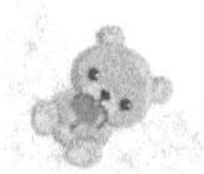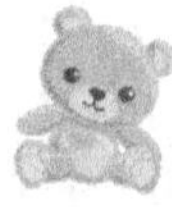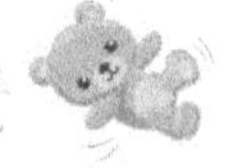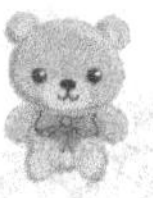

"No kids, it won't. Boats have a special engine to go fast and carry on with the car's weight."

The ferry had a huge mouth where the cars drove in and, from my view, it looked like it was swallowing each one slowly, one by one, like a giant monster. We approached the police control where a few men with serious faces were checking documents, tickets and stuff. I didn't really know what they were, nor did I understand a word they were saying. It sounded like they were mumbling from where I was sitting, but Mamita told us they were policemen.

It was the first time in my life travelling in such a huge boat. I'd sailed in my daddy's old red one, which always ended up stopping in the middle of nowhere because of some engine failure; whenever that happened, he fixed it so we could return to the coast. Can you imagine?

The moment we got to enter, the music was at full blast. It sounded like we were in a movie scene, screaming, jumping on the car seats super excited, recording videos. Once inside, there were people showing us the way to our parking spot: the giant's belly. We got out carrying only the necessary items to our rooms, which, on the ships, were called "cabins". The parking lot inside the ship smelled like the sea and dead fish. There was also water pooling on the floor, and I hoped our car wouldn't get completely wet.

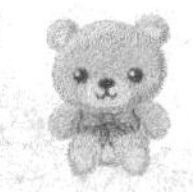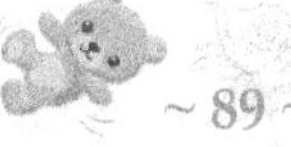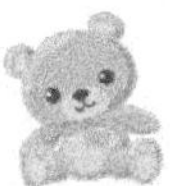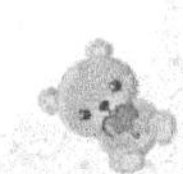

"Mamita, lock the car and roll up the windows tightly so that no water gets in."

"Yes princess, don't worry, I've closed everything very well. It won't get wet, trust me."

We headed to an elevator and several people entered at once with their bags and suitcases. At the reception level, the boat staff gave us the keys to our cabin.

"Oh, this looks like a hotel, it's nothing like my daddy's little boat! It's so nice in here!"

It had carpets everywhere! Lots of fancy hallways! Four or five levels!

'How can a boat have so many levels and so many elevators?' I kept thinking to myself in awe and wonder.

There was also a wide staircase like a palace, and a corridor with many room doors, all of them identical. Ours was right in the middle and Mamita opened it using a weird card she slid through a slot. I was fascinated on seeing it work.

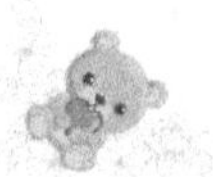 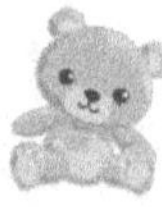 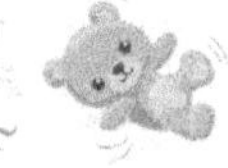 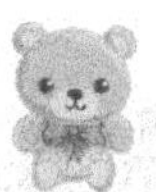

I kept wondering if it truly was boat. It felt like a building. Our cabin had four beds, two at the top and two at the bottom, a tiny table in between, and a bathroom with a shower… so nice! It really was like a hotel room! I couldn't help playing with the cabin key, closing and opening the door with the card once again. I was trying to discover how it worked but it seemed way too complicated.

We heard the hum of the engines as they started. Hooray! We were moving through the water with the whole building and a bunch of cars inside! The boys and I were running around the ferry, watching the boat glide through the waters and enter the ocean.

"Going out to sea is called sailing. I mean, we're sailing now," Klim told us.

"How do you know that?" I asked him.

"I read a book about ships, and plus, I've seen movies."

'What an odd word, "sail". I know the word "saving", but "sailing"?' It was stuck in my mind.

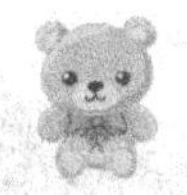 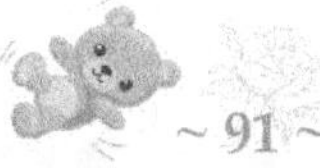 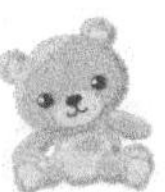 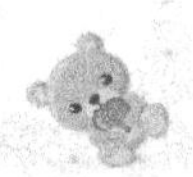

It was really windy outside on deck and we had so much fun exploring the boat from top to bottom. There were lots of restaurants, even a movie theater! But Mamita said we couldn't go to any of them because they were too expensive. It was all right. We had food that she'd bought at the supermarket back on Roscoff, so eating in the cabin was cool too. For a moment, we'd forgotten where our room was and had a hard time finding it since all the doors were alike on every single level. I was relieved when we found it. That was scary!

The top bed had removable metal stairs. So Klim pulled out two and turned them over, placing the hooks down so they looked like legs; then he climbed up to the middle and tried to walk, like a clown. We laughed out loud because it gave the illusion that he had long legs.

We traveled all night, and the boat was moving quickly. Mommy and Klim felt sick. They said it was seasickness, and that it happened to some people. Pavel and I were fine, so Mamita sent us to a store to buy some bracelets; she said they had a bracelet that, when worn by the person, squeezed a vein on your wrist. Even though we brought it right away, Mami and Klim didn't feel any better, and it seemed the bracelet was not very helpful. There was no other choice but to wait until we reached our destination. We had to hold on for the night.

We finally made it to the shore.

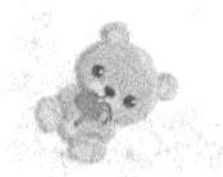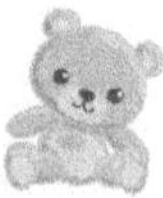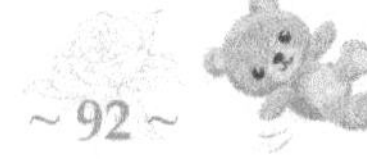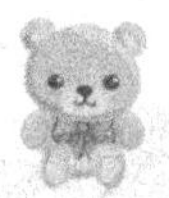

"We're getting there! We're sailing, sailing!" I screamed out to learn the new word.

"Actually, Katerina, we are mooring." Klim corrected. "We're not sailing… sailing is when the ship comes out of the port, and mooring is when the ship arrives."

"Ugh. How many names, Klim?" I asked. "Isn't it easier to say go and come?"

"You think you're a brainiac?" Pavel asked him.

"Obviously!" Klim replied smugly.

We couldn't wait to get permission to leave for our car. I kept hoping it hadn't sunk. The moment the huge gates were opened, so much water rushed through it. Once again, the nasty smell of sea and dead fish permeated the air. I was sure the car had gotten wet.

"Mami! Are you sure our car is okay, Mamita?"

"I hope so, honey," she answered, and it seemed to me she wasn't so sure either. After all, it was her first time traveling by boat too.

I was a bit scared when we were finally able to go down to the garage. The smell of dead fish was too strong, but our car was still where we'd left it. It hadn't gotten wet at all. Phew. Thank God.

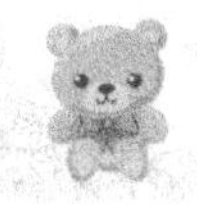 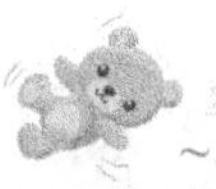 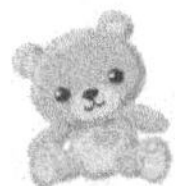 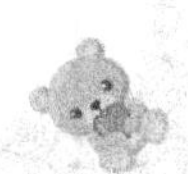

"Katerina, get off!" Klim suddenly yelled at me. "We're landing!"

"Great! We're landing!" I repeated.

"Say "Hi" to Cork City, guys! We're in Ireland now!" Mamita announced happily. "We're going to drive a bit more and take a look at the houses on the way."

We said goodbye to the boat, and showed our appreciation to it for having crossed the ocean without sinking.

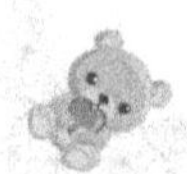 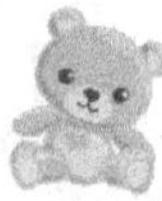 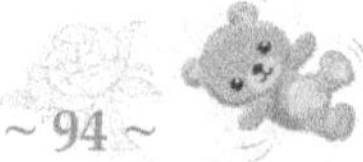 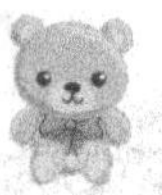

IRELAND

Ireland is surely a peculiar place. I notice that the cars are being driven on the other side of the road. Plus, it seems like summer is already over in this country because it's raining when we arrive, and the people seem to be wearing multiple layers of clothes. Mamita has to drive a thousand more hours to our first stop in the city of Carrik-On-Shannon. So, in the meantime, Klim and I have fun using the lilac colored sheet as if it were a hut.

"Knock, knock! Can I come in?" Klim asks, pretending there's a door.

"Yes! Come in, Klim," I answer. And so on we play, until we get bored.

We make it to the first house where there's lush grass and cows everywhere. A lady shows us around, and although it is beautiful, it's also empty and cold. So mamita doesn't like it very much and tells us we better go visit the next one, but on our second stop, it's the same thing.

Third stop: Charlestown. We like the city a lot more since there are far less cows and more people. Someone shows us the house and I believe we all fell in love with it.

Klim's the first to speak up. "Mommy, shall we stay here? We like it, don't we?"

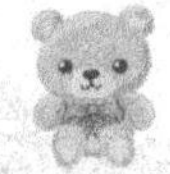
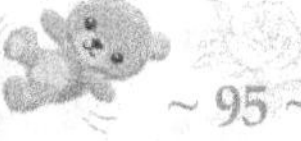
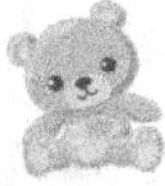
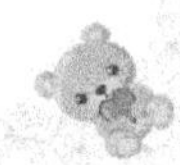

"Yes, mamita! The house is beauuutiful!" I agree with him.

"Yeah, it's pretty nice," Mami finally says.

"What about Donegal's house, mom? That one we saw in the pictures?" Pavel asks. "We liked it a lot too! Maybe that house is better, don't you think?"

"Yes, honey. Actually, you're right. I know you're tired, kids, but that one seems to be on the top of the list. Let's take a look."

"Okay," Klim and I reply dejected, with no desire to go anywhere else. Although we like both the house and the city, we'll be continuing our journey.

Mami stops at a mini-market on the way, looking for some iced tea; she finds something that's similar to the one we usually buy in Spain, but when we open the bottle, some weird gas pops out.

"Oops, that's strange...it's got gas! What is this, mommy?" Klim asks her.

"I don't know guys, let's find out."

We take a sip and EW! It's not like the stuff we normally get.

"It's disgusting! It tastes really bad!"

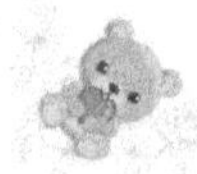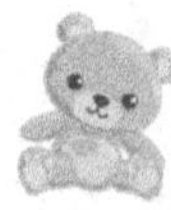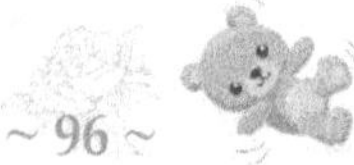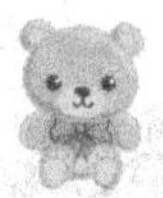

"Yes, it's terrible," my mommy agrees. In the end, we don't have to throw it away because Pavel likes it.

We then drive to an even bigger city, with no cows, but many, many beautiful buildings and houses. Donegal is awesome! I feel like our new home might be here. Since it's located to the north of the island, it's even colder than the other places we've been to. The moment we arrive in a very nice area, a woman gives us a signal from her car, so we follow her; all of the houses are really big and lovely, all of them, except… WHAT?

The lady turns into a narrow and muddy road, and my mommy began to complain, "Ooh! What is this?"

We see a strange, creepy, ugly and twisted witch hideaway – or, at least, it seems like it; where there should have been a path, there's only mud with a wooden plank on top for us to cross. The place is awful but we decide to give it a try and see the inside. I don't like this house, and I don't need to go inside to know that.

Luckily, mamita seems to have read my mind because everything in the house has been placed upside down. So, she says something to the woman that I can't really understand, then turns around and informs us, "Let's get out of here, fast! This house is definitely not for us!" she says in Russian, and we run away following her instructions.

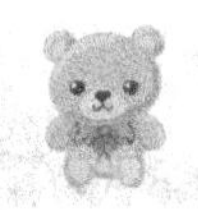 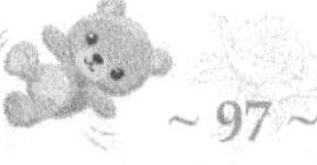 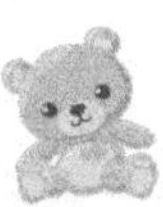 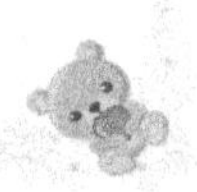

We continue the endless journey, but now I don't know where we are going and it's beginning to get dark. I think there's another house on the list, so my mommy calls the owners and then drives there. We arrive late at night, exhausted, but we've finally found a place to stay. The house is huge, with six rooms and a big TV in the living area. I think that's the reason why Pavel likes it so bad. That's it! We'll be keeping the house. I stay with mami in the largest room, and I'm so sleepy that I fall asleep right away.

Our first night in a foreign country? Check. I'm immediately hungry once we wake up! In the morning, my mommy prepares a nice breakfast, and even though the food here tastes different, she manages to make it delicious, as always. There's only one shower, so Pavel, Klim and I compete for the first turn to take a bath. We get ready to go out and take a look at the city and the schools, but since my big brother is still in the shower, Klim and I watch cartoons on TV until he finishes. I can only pay attention to what the characters are doing because I don't understand what they're saying. They speak too fast and the language sounds very strange to me.

Here in Ireland, everyone speaks English. The TV doesn't have even a single channel in Spanish, and despite understanding more than I do, Klim doesn't want to translate anything for me. As we are still waiting for Pavel, mommy suddenly screams from the kitchen, "Oh no, not that!"

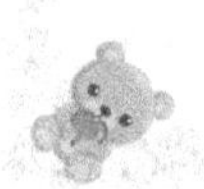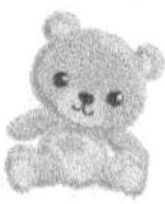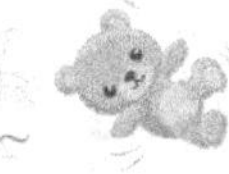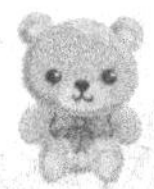

We get there as fast as we can, and find her looking up at the ceiling. So we turn our gazes up and find… it's raining through a hole in the ceiling!

"We can't stay in this house since we can't repair it. Who is going to help us here?"

Mommy runs to the shower and tells Pavel to get out quickly. "We can't stay in this house, son. It's leaking and the pipes seem to be old and rotten…" she explains everything to him.

My big brother's mood changes quickly, from being scared to getting angry, as soon as he hears that. He doesn't like the idea of leaving; nevertheless, Klim and I are happy, but we have to stay silent so Pavel doesn't get any more upset. Even though the owners arrive and offer mommy some repairs, she decides we'll be going back to Charlestown, to the house we liked more. Woohoo!

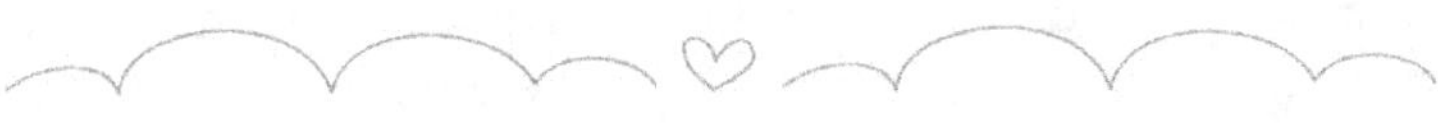

OUR NEW HOME IN CHARLESTOWN

"We have a home, kids! You can choose the rooms you want to keep," Mommy says, after receiving the keys from the owners, who leave immediately.

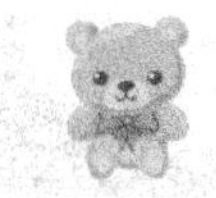
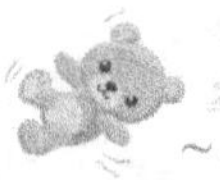
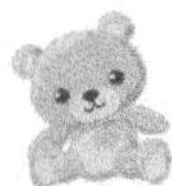
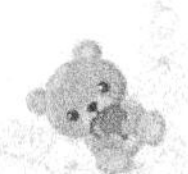

She's referring to the boys since I have the privilege of staying in the big room with her. This house is warmer than the others, and way cozier. We run upstairs and then downstairs, trying to figure out where everything is. It's fantastic to have a new home. Finally!

The first floor has a living room with nice furniture and a wide fireplace, but no TV, unfortunately. On the other hand, the kitchen is much bigger and has a large glass door that leads you to the backyard with a beautiful garden. The lovely garden is lush with green grass and is surrounded by a wooden fence. There's so many kitties walking around.

On the second floor, there's three rooms with double beds and three bathrooms. Our room is bigger than my brothers' and even has its own bathroom with a shower. The boys' bathroom is by the hall and has a bathtub instead.

Mamita tells us that we can buy everything we need, but first, we'll need to rest a little bit. The break turns into a couple of days without going anywhere. Fortunately, there is a supermarket behind this neighborhood where we can buy some food. We eat, sleep, eat, sleep, and repeat, until mamita finally regains her energy to go out.

One morning, she tells us, "We are going shopping in a bigger city, with lots of stores."

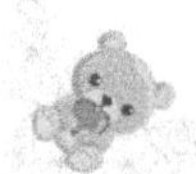 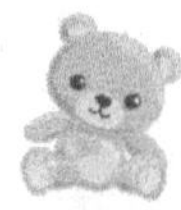 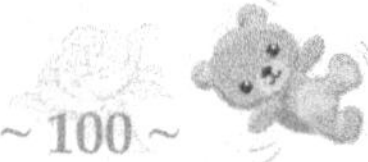 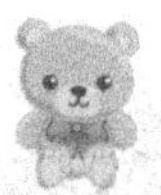

Now we will have beddings, great! No more jackets, T-shirts and stockings to cover ourselves! Oh! And mami could also buy me some panties for my size!

We leave home early and drive to Castlebar, the closest and biggest town. There are several stores and supermarkets where we buy food, bedding (especially some thick blankets to keep us warm at night), spoons, forks, knives…

And then some more clothes, pillows, utensils, soaps, toothpaste, brushes, towels and I don't know what else. Oh! And of course, my panties! In the end, mami buys so much stuff that the car doesn't have enough space, so we are loaded to the brim, up to the ceiling. I can hardly breathe. I can't even see my brother next to me, or mommy and Pavel in the front seats… I really want to get home, now.

DISCOVERING CHARLESTOWN

As our new life in Ireland begins, we start going out to discover everything around us, especially the location of the schools. We connect with the family in Spain via. video call and show them the place.

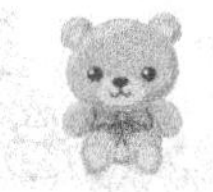 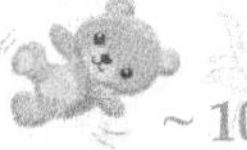 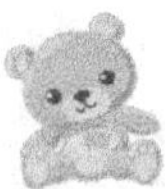 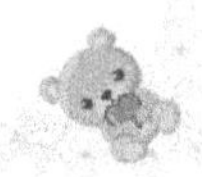

It is a ten-minute walk from the house to downtown. We also discover bars, hairdressers, drugstores, restaurants and a church on the way. We even find a library. Mami finds someone to talk to, but since they speak in English, I don't understand a word they say. But I guess it is about the schools because the man points to where they are, and then we go in that direction. My school is pretty small; it has only one level. I'm going to be start my fourth year of primary school at St. Attracta's.

A little further ahead is the secondary school where Pavel and Klim will be going. It's called St. Joseph's, and it's much bigger and nicer... I like it better.

There is also a big kid's park near my school, with swings, trampolines, ropes, slides and other fun things, like a soccer field. We run to the swings the moment we see them, it's so much fun! It'd be nice to talk to some of the children here, but I don't understand them, and they wouldn't understand me either. What weird kids.

There's also a basketball court next to the park, and behind the soccer field is a cemetery. That's not really nice at all, but thank God for the huge church. It's very beautiful and looks like something out of an old movie

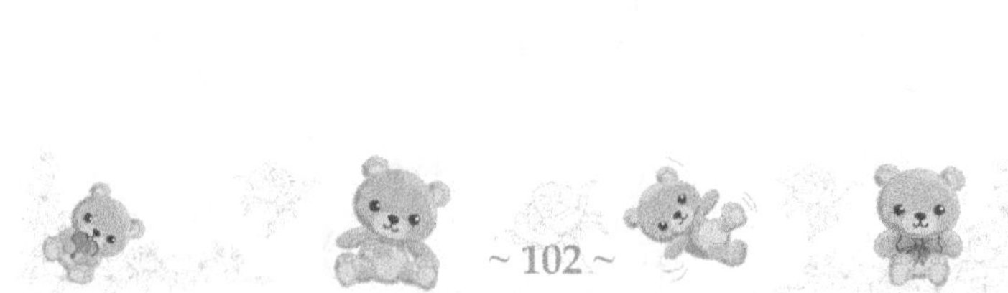

NEW SCHOOL

The kids in Charlestown have to wear uniforms for school. I've never worn something like that before, but I really like the one I have to wear. It's a black skirt paired with a white shirt, and a gray sweater with the green school crest on the right side of my chest. Actually, it is better than the striped gown I used to wear during recess at Ignaci Iglesias.

The boys have a more elegant uniform. Their sweater is a nice color, a mix between brown and red (mami told me it's called "burgundy"), with the school's crest in yellow, a light blue shirt underneath, and dark gray pants. The shoes have to be black and no sneakers are allowed.

How cool! Looks like we're going to Hogwarts!

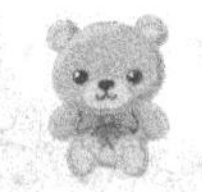
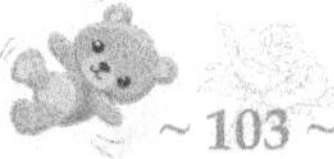
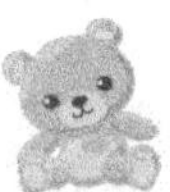
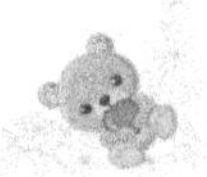

I am excited, but a bit nervous on our first day of school. Everyone is starting to line up and I'm not sure where I'm supposed to go, or anything at all, but I calm down as soon as I see Mrs. Reilly. She is a teacher who mamita had introduced me to, at a meeting, so I get in that line; she spots me and greets me with a big smile, then introduces me to a classmate named Shona. It's so amazing I'll have new friends! This girl will be teaching me school things for the first few months, or, until I get used to the language. She's some kind of a "buddy" – kids who accompany the new students so they don't get lost or feel lonely. When we get to the classroom, both the third- and fourth-class children are in the same room. Schools in Ireland are pretty different.

'How are we going to study like this? Do I have to learn two levels at a time?' I ask myself, curious.

Schools in Spain are much more crowded and the buildings are huge. Here, it doesn't look so much like a school, but more like a big house with a big family. I don't know if that's better or worse, but it just doesn't feel the same. My mommy explained to me that since the city isn't that big, there's not enough students to teach separate classes.

Mrs. Reilly shows me where I should sit. Although I don't understand what she says, I understand what she means by her gestures, so I do.

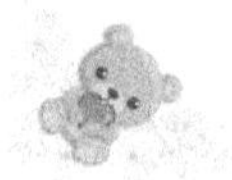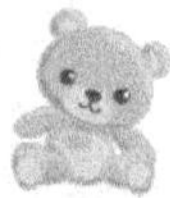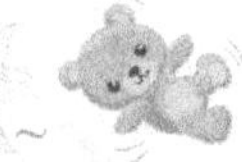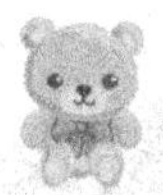

Every day, I feel more and more at home here. I had a good time at the apartment we used to live in in Barcelona, but I like our new, giant house better. In Ireland, it is constantly raining…well, not that much, but almost; plus, everything in this country is so bright green, that it even hurts my eyes! I love that everything here looks like toys – like the little houses downtown, painted in different colors like dolls'. The scenery is very different from Barcelona with its huge buildings, and the blue Mediterranean sea. We're enjoying getting to know the other nearby cities on weekends… It's like a fairytale here

TRIP TO SPAIN

Mámachka tells us that "Make a Wish" just called. It seems they want to take us to Disneyland in Paris, even though I'd said I didn't want to, and she'd accepted. Now that I've seen our new home, I want a new adventure as well. I think it'd be fun to go to that park. The best thing is that we can make a quick trip to Spain, and since it's already September, I'm going to have a great time celebrating my birthday with all my family together! With no school, by the way. Isn't it perfect?

Our bags are packed and ready to go, and so are we. We wake up early because Olga, a new Russian friend of

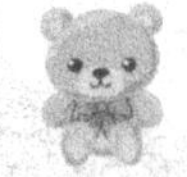
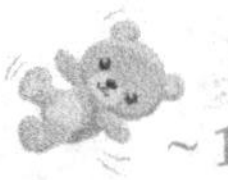
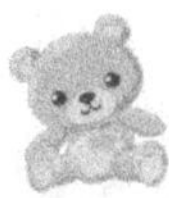
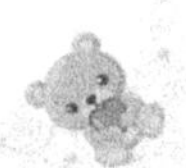

Mami's, is going to take us to the airport, which is really close to Charlestown. So, we are heading there. I'm impressed! I've never been in a plane like this before, or looked at the planes from up close. In fact, it's my first flight ever!

At the airport, after first checking in, an agent of some kind hands us the tickets and we drop off the bigger bags. I don't understand why, but those are the rules.

"They put them in a space at the bottom of the plane, sweetie, and when we land, they are going to give them back to us," Mamita explains to me.

For the next step, we go to the checkpoints where some long-faced people in uniform make us take off our shoes and pass through a bow; we also have to leave our bags and coats on trays that pass through a tunnel, and wait for them on the other side.

We stand in front of some huge windows where you can see the planes from up close; they look like something out of a movie. My brothers are very happy too. They were pretty small during their first air travel, when they arrived in Spain from Russia… but I'd still been inside mamita's belly, so I don't remember that trip.

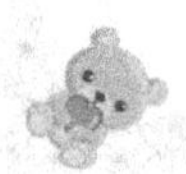
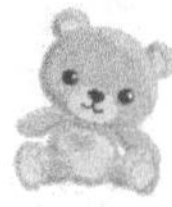
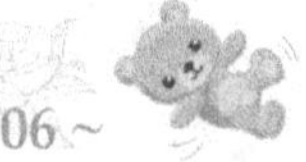
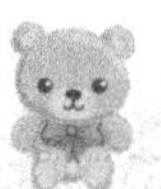

The boarding begins and we walk outside to get to the plane, which is way bigger than I'd thought it would be. It is very windy, so my hair is out of control. The experience gives me so much joy that I shout out of happiness.

"Look! Look how big it is!"

There is a line of people waiting to get on the plane using a very steep metal ladder. My mommy tells me, "This plane is not so big… it is very small, actually."

I cannot imagine something bigger than this, where I feel like thousands of Katerinas can fit in.

We take several photos before getting on board.

"We won't fly for too long since plane travels are faster than road trips," my mommy says.

We each take our places and fasten our seatbelts, while the flight attendants teach us some rules in case of an emergency, making funny signs with her hands. The engine starts making a loud noise that reminds me of rockets. It starts going faster and faster until suddenly it starts rising into the air. We're flying! For real! As the plane takes off, the ground looks like it's moving farther and farther away, while the people and buildings get smaller and smaller. WOW! I can't stay quiet… my heart is racing while I look through the round window.

As we get higher and higher into the air, the plane starts trembling. I feel like throwing up. Plus, there's some kind of pressure inside my ears. So mamita tells us that we should fill our cheeks with air, explaining how to blow without opening our mouths, but it doesn't come out; we just look like hamsters. She insists on her instructions and after many, many tries, I can hear clearly again.

Wow! Now the plane is moving so smoothly, I can hardly feel it. It even gives the impression of it standing still on the ground. My brothers and I immediately stick our faces to the windows, pushing each other, as soon as we are allowed to unbuckle our seatbelts.

The city is now gone… there's only a toy town. Plus, we are flying among the clouds, literally! I imagine they are giant absorbent cotton chunks, and that I can jump or sleep on them. They seem so soft and yummy that I ask mamita, "Can you jump in these clouds?"

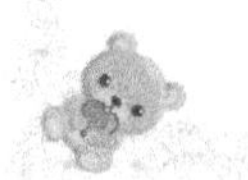 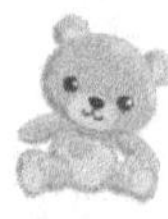 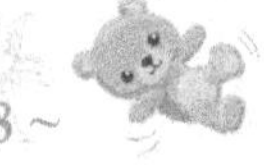 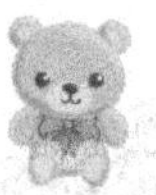

"No baby," she says sweetly. "They are like… white air, you know? As a thick fog, like when you can't see anything, it's the same. The clouds can't hold weight, you would pass through them."

I listen to my mommy but I keep thinking she can't know because she has never tried it. If mami gives it a try, she would see how soft they are.

After a while, we fly through the clouds and the outside turns blurry, so looking through the window is no longer fun. My brothers and I start walking around, investigating what's here and there. We find two mini bathrooms and my curiosity makes me go inside. Somehow, I accidentally end up locking it, but manage to get out and run back to *mámachka*. I ask her to come with me the second time. When we get there, I press the toilet button and the water sounds like a vacuum cleaner.

I ask her, "Mamita! Mami, where do things go from the toilet? Do they go through the air and fall on people?

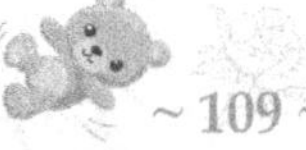
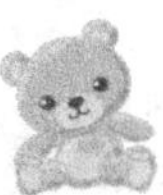
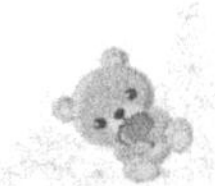

"No honey," she giggles. "There's a tank underneath the plane where they fall in. The airport staff take it out when we land, and change it for the next flight," she explains patiently to me. "Otherwise it would be disgusting to have poop fall on you out of nowhere, right?"

"Right. We would always have to carry an umbrella in case it falls. Yuck!"

"Exactly," Mamita laughs.

The flight attendant is asking us to buckle up, so we go back to our seats, but we are not so happy about it. I get anxious about the landing. The plane starts making a lot of noise, and as we starting going down, my ears are blocked, again. Suddenly BAM! I think we've run into some aliens, but mamita immediately clarifies what really happened, "It's the wheels of the plane that touched the ground."

I feel my head is going to explode from a crash like that. The plane moves fast, but eventually starts slowing down, until it finally stops.

"We are already in Spain!" my mommy exclaims with excitement.

I can't wait to get out. It's weird that we arrived in Spain in such a short time. We flew for about three hours, but

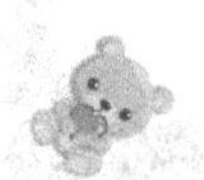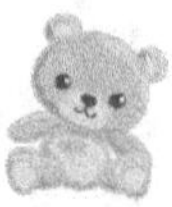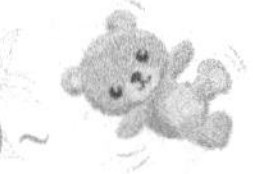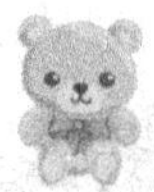

time went by so fast, it didn't feel real. If I remember right, the road trip to Ireland seemed endless. Mamita spent too many nights driving, while Klim, Pavel and I ate and slept.

The moment we get out of the plane, I feel the warm Spanish weather. Is it possible that I have already forgotten what the heat is like here? We haven't been in the green country for too long, but I believe I'm used to the cold there by now.

At the Reus' Airport, my uncle Ilusha is waiting to take us to my granny's house.

"Babulia!"

We get to my granny's in a few minutes and I run to her arms as soon as I see her.

"Vnúchenka!"

She hugs me tightly, and then she greets my mommy and brothers. *"Privet moi dorogíe vnuchata! Privet dóchenka! How quickly you arrived! I've missed you!"*

"We missed you too, babulia!"

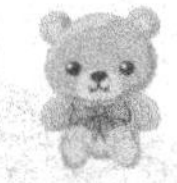 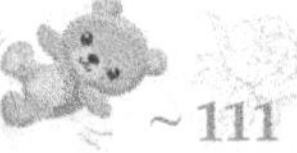 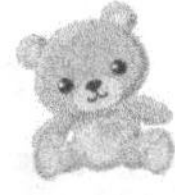 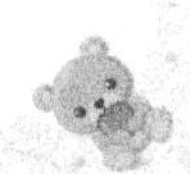

I'm happy to see my family again. We get excited talking about Ireland and the trip during the whole afternoon.

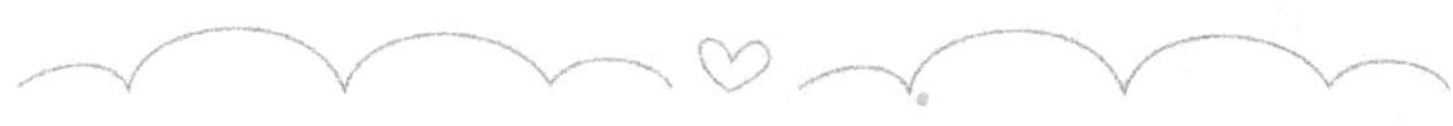

A DREAM SURPRISE!

We head for Barcelona to the "Make a Wish" office, where they'll be giving us the tickets for the Disneyland trip. Soon I will get to know Rapunzel and Tiana, my favorite princesses of all time. Rapunzel is blonde with green eyes, and has a long magical braid that's thousands of meters long. Princess Tiana is a brunette, who wears a super beautiful dress that makes her look like a flower; her boyfriend is a handsome prince, and their story is the cutest – an evil wizard turned him into a frog with a spell. At first, Tiana didn't want to kiss him, but in the end, he convinced her, and she turned into a frog too. What a mess! I guess it's not easy being a frog.

My daddy is driving us and since he loves taking pictures, he brings his camera with him. I am happy because the company promised me that I will see the princesses who live beyond this world, in a kingdom far, far away; maybe they will cross the most mysterious oceans and forests to meet me in Paris.

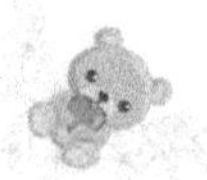 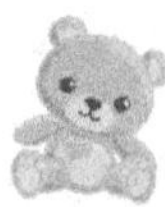 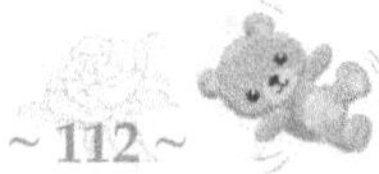 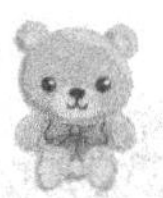

Here we are, and Lourdes gives us a warm welcome in her office. She then invites us to take a seat inside a huge room and says, "Hi everyone! Katerina, we are happy we can now help you make your dream come true. Are you ready for Disneyland?"

"Yes!" I respond, with joy.

Lourdes gives me a huge catalog with a drawing on the cover. It has my name, along with the Make-a-Wish foundation's too. I already know how to read well. My mommy taught me when I was five years old.

"Open the first page, Katerina, and take a look where you will be going," she tells me.

 I open the colorful notebook very carefully to see what's inside, and there's a big map with a tiny plane on it. No doubt I'll be going on a trip by plane.

Lourdes asks me again, "Where are you going, Katerina? Where are you taking your family?"

I don't really know what she means, nor do I understand much about maps... Besides, mommy already told me where we'll be going, so why does she keep asking me that?

"To Disneyland!" I answer, without thinking too much.

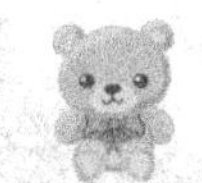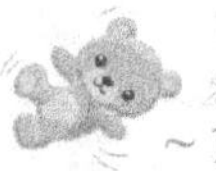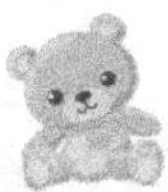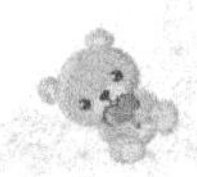

"Take a good look at the map, baby girl," Lourdes continues. "Take a good look at it, where are you going?"

I find it to be a very weird question since I'm sure she knows perfectly well where they want me to go with my family, so I tell her, "To Paris!"

Everyone stares at me, giggling, and Lourdes keeps asking me over and over again.

"Pay attention to the notebook. Where are you going, Katerina? Look at the map closely. What route does the plane show on the map?"

I check it out, once again... it's marked with dots, but I don't get it. What am I supposed to see? I try to think harder about my answer so they understand me.

"To France, to Disneyland!"

All of them smile at me and I smile back. I think I finally answered it right, but then I notice my brothers are a bit nervous; Klim is sweating and rubbing his hands, while Pavel has an ear-to-ear grin on his face. It looks like they want to say something, which is not helpful at all. I give up. I don't know what else I can answer.

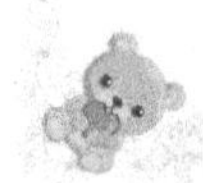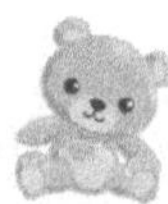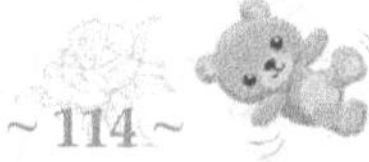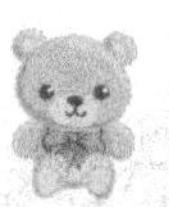

"Dóchenka, do you remember you wanted to visit the princesses' castles, the real ones? Look at the map again; look at it carefully. Do you remember when we traveled from Spain to Ireland by car – first I drove all across France and there was no water in between? Look, there is Ireland," my mommy points out on the map to me. "Do you see that we crossed the ocean just a little bit? Look at the map. The plane is flying over lots and lots of water. Much further. That can't be France, right? I mean, that country is not that far from here, plus there's no water at all. Take a good look."

That's true. I look at the map one more time, and when I see such a huge amount of water, I realize that it must be farther from Paris. Then I read "American Continent", where I'd really wanted to go…

'What? Am I really getting it right?' I ask myself. I cannot believe it! I cannot answer the question to mommy, or Lourdes. What if I'm wrong? I don't know much geography.

 Maybe Lourdes read my mind because she looks at me and says, "Isn't Florida where you wanted to go? Does it look like it's where you're going to take your family, Katerina? You're going to Orlando!

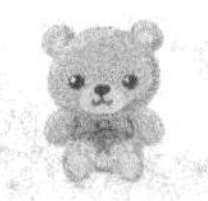
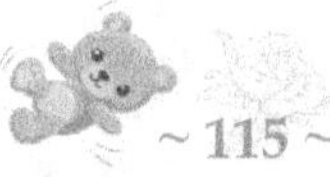
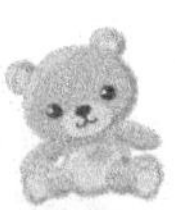
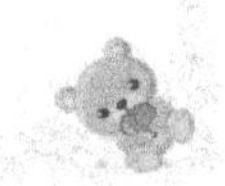

I look at Lourdes, then at my mommy, and as I see their happy faces, I realize they're not joking. We're going to America! I still can't believe it. Is my dream going to come true? I cover my eyes with my hands and start crying emotionally, louder and louder. Lourdes immediately leans towards me and we hug tightly.

Once I calm down a bit and take a look around, I notice everyone's crying too; my mommy, my daddy, my brothers... seeing their faces soaked in tears of happiness, I can't keep from crying loudly again. It's such a magical day, I'm so happy.

"Let's see Katerina, how is your trip going to be? Open the next page," Lourdes tells me.

The whole trip is marked. Where we are going to stay, who will be receiving us at each stop, how we are going to travel, the places we are going to visit and who we are going to meet... Everything is here!

"There will be many surprises!" she continues.

'What other surprises? More than this seems impossible!' I think to myself.

I hug mamita tightly and try to concentrate on what the adults are talking about, but there's only one word in my head – joy, joy, joy, joy, joy again and so on, and forth; that's all I can think about right now, but I know both my mom and my brothers will explain everything later.

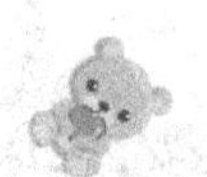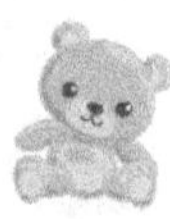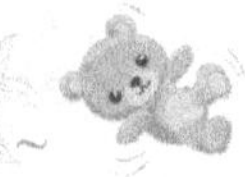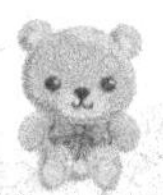

Lourdes hands us the passports with some super long tickets and a package, then she turns around to tell me, "Congratulations Katerina! Your dream is about to come true! Mickey and Minnie Mouse really liked your projects and they decided to give you this opportunity. So when you get there, make sure to give them a huge hug.

Enjoy the trip, and don't forget to take a bunch of pictures to show us and tell us all about the adventure! We wish you the best of luck!" I feel very special because I know they love me.

We leave the building really excited; how could mami keep such a secret? How could she hide the truth? My brothers don't stop hugging me and ask mommy, "Mommy! Mommy, how did you do it? Why didn't you tell us anything?"

"If I had told you, it wouldn't be such a surprise for everyone, right?" she answers, and we shout with enjoyment and hug each other. I still can't believe my dream will come true! How is it possible? I feel so happy, I don't want to even think about the possibilities. I just want to go there right now!

The return home is very enthusiastic, and we pack everything for our trip to the USA on the other side of the planet. Humans don't travel there – it's a magic kingdom where all of my favorite princesses live.

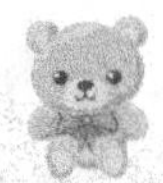
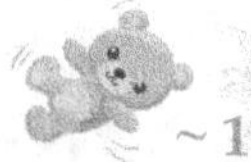
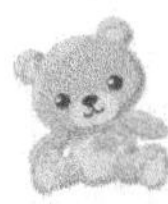
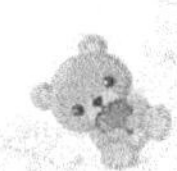

TRIP TO ORLANDO

All our bags are packed, and this time, Oso is going with me. I haven't named him yet, but he's still my big brown faithful friend. We will be together during this charmed trip which neither he, nor anyone else, has experienced. Mine is a different story since I'm not a regular girl…I am magical.

My daddy arrives early in the morning to give us a ride to the airport in Barcelona. Once there, we see our guide waiting at the entrance with a huge smile. He explains that we'll first be going to Madrid, then another flight will take us to New York, and lastly to Orlando, Florida. After checking the passports at the registration table, the people there wish us a great journey and take our bags to a conveyor. This is the second time I'll be travelling this way and I feel like an expert because, by now, I understand some stuff that back in the time seemed strange to me.

The guide leads us to a luxurious room called the VIP area, that has many beautiful and comfortable seats, soft sofas, small tables, and a free buffet to choose whatever we want to eat. A few fancy ladies in heels and teacher's clothes bring us gifts and yummy snacks for the trip; they were sent to attend to us by Iberia, the company we'll be flying with.

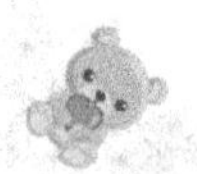 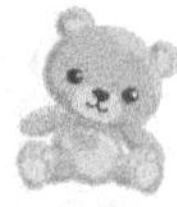 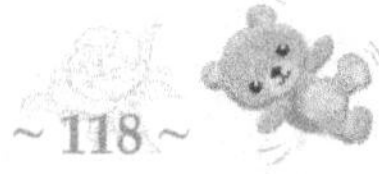 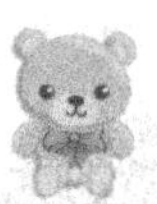

I think the line we're standing in is also special, since we will be the first to go inside, and there's almost no one in this line. Anyways, once we get inside the plane, we are greeted by the good-looking stewardesses of this flight, wearing matching red scarves on their necks, and a weird red cap.

"Welcome to our flight! Have a seat!"

They offer to let us see the cockpit, but I think that's more of a boy thing. My brothers get very excited and go to take a look, while I give the pilots the thank you letter we wrote at home.

"Thank you so much, Katerina, it's truly beautiful," they say after reading it.

We wrote letters for all the pilots who will be taking us to Disneyworld. I drew many faces with googly eyes on them, which they liked a lot. The pilots answer our questions, let us sit in their seats and touch every single button above and below the window, and even a few between the seats…

"How do you remember what each button is for?" I ask. "There are thousands of them!"

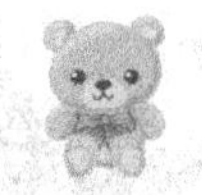
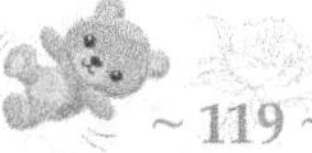
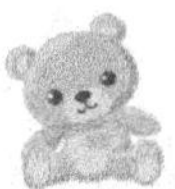
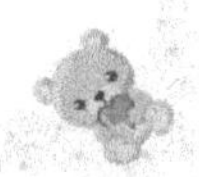

"Well, we don't always remember, but there's a whole team helping us from the ground." I know they aren't telling me the truth because, come on, they must know what each button is for, or we would all crash or something.

My brothers don't stop asking them how to speed up, and many other things I don't really listen to since I'm already disconnected from all the questions. The pilot's seat is so comfy that I don't care about anything else.

We return to our seats and wait for take-off, and soon, the clouds are among us. The elegant ladies bring us drinks and munchies, so I wonder: is this the life of a princess? I feel like it is, definitely. Before landing, we are called back to the cockpit.

"Would you like to see the plane land from here?"

"Yes! Yes! Yes! Of course!" We jumped up from the seats in excitement. *"Of course we want to see it!"*

The pilots communicate with the people working on the ground through microphones, like in the movies; they press a lot of buttons, then move the levers from one side to the other… They do so many things that I am pretty alarmed, not understanding how they don't make any mistakes.

"Look, we are going to land soon!" They shake me out of my thoughts.

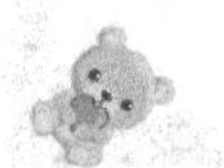
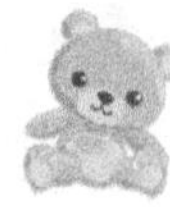
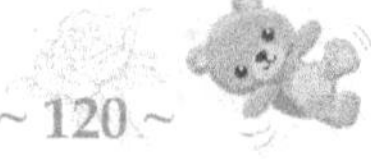
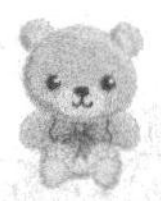

"Where? We want to see everything."

Watching the plane landing from this point of view is a whole completely different experience, than seeing it from the small round window for the passengers. Here, the earth looks much more beautiful as we approach it. In the end, once we touch the runway, the landing make us jump in our seats. It felt like we'd crashed into the ground.

"Cool! This is so much fun!" we applaud joyfully.

The boys and I go back to our places since we're supposed to get out of the plane first, and the staff won't let anyone else leave until that happens. We see a few ladies on the other side of the gate waiting to greet us.

"Welcome to Madrid, Katerina, welcome everyone!" They say with a smile on their faces.

WOW! They know me here too! Am I famous?

"Your plane for New York is waiting for you. We need to run, Katerina, they're about to take off but they can't leave without you."

We take a small train inside the airport while they explain our next steps, flights, and many other things; they also give us yellow T-shirts with the words "Maagic Flight" printed on them, which we have to wear until the final trip to Orlando. It's a kind of identification for the people who will be receiving us there.

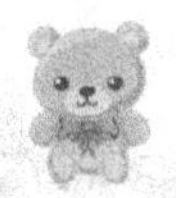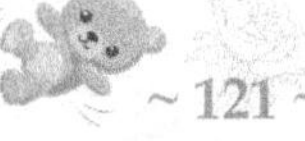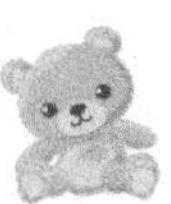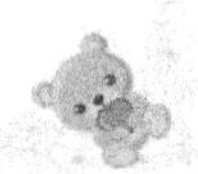

After the train ride is over, we run fast through some long corridors, and my sandal breaks during the hustle. So I keep running without shoes since there's no time to find stores nearby to buy them. The floor is cold, but I don't complain. Mamita stops for a moment and takes her flip-flops out of her suitcase for me; even though they're too big for my feet, I like wearing them. I feel more like an adult. The thing is, that running in these is not easy at all; my feet get tangled up and I fall down. Besides, Oso feels quite heavy from carrying it for so long, but I keep running as fast as I can, along with everyone else.

Thank God the plane is still waiting for us! The ladies give me a card with money that I can use at the parks, and to buy gifts. Then we say goodbye and board the adventure of crossing the ocean. My mommy constantly keeps showing us the booklet Lourdes had given us, so now I have a very clear image of how we'll be flying over miles and miles of water.

This plane makes the one in Ireland seem like a toy… it's as huge as a spaceship! Not huge… GIANT! As we enter, two flight attendants wearing bright red lipstick greet us. They also wear matching blue clothes, and heels. Their uniform is actually similar to the ones from the last plane we were in, but in different colors.

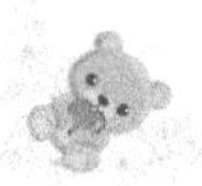 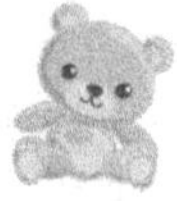 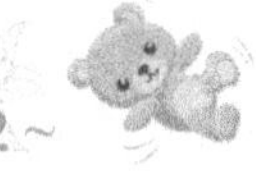 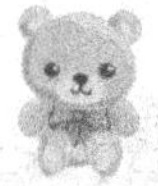

Everyone starts applauding, whistling and shouting my name "Katerina, Katerina, welcome!" I get a bit scared and grab onto my mommy's skirt, whispering in a quieter voice in Russian, so nobody can hear or understand us.

"Mommy! Mommy, how do they know my name? How do they know who I am? I don't know anyone here."

"You are very famous, sweetheart. This trip is yours and since you're the princess, everybody knows you."

At first, it feels a bit weird that suddenly everybody knows me and I don't know anyone here. I can feel all the attention on me and actually, it's scary. Nevertheless, during the journey, I start feeling more relaxed with all the love they give me. In fact, I don't feel like a princess at all, but a queen.

My brothers and I are invited to the cockpit once again; this one is bigger, and has more buttons. The pilots in this flight are North Americans, so they only speak English. It's a good thing I have Pavel and Klim to translate everything they say so that I can understand them, even if it's just a bit...

Still, I keep answering "Yes" to every question they ask me. I know they like the letter we gave them because they look happy and give me a big hug.

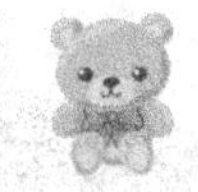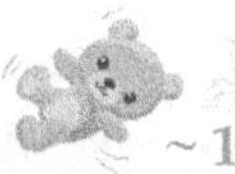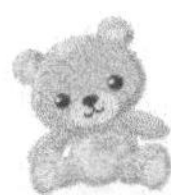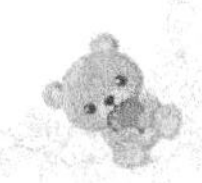

During takeoff, as we return to our seats, I notice that this plane is so long that it looks like a sausage – there's an aisle on both sides, separated by an extra seating row in the middle. It's endless.

I can see Madrid through the window, with its tall buildings gradually becoming smaller like toys as we rise higher into the air. The people also look like tiny living dolls, and all I want is to put them in my pocket to play with them later when I'm back home, but the plane's doors are locked and I can't get out.

The clouds draw close to the windows again, and I keep thinking about their softness; surely we could sleep or jump over them if adults weren't such spoilsports. At some point, I feel like throwing up and my ears are clogged up again, but this time, I succeed in using the technique that mamita had taught us, so I clear them perfectly.

The moment the seatbelt light disappears, we get up and run around seeing all the places we could, and those that we shouldn't, too; however, we soon get tired and look for our seats, which I thought had disappeared since it took us a while to find them. However, I calm down when we finally do.

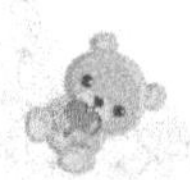
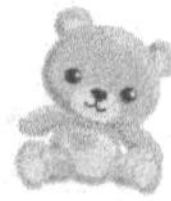
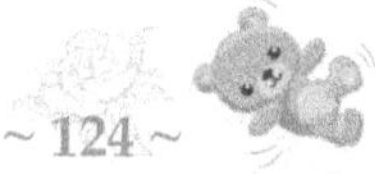
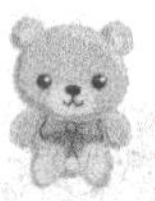

Something smells delicious and they begin serving some nice meals similar to a restaurant…or, nope, more like an alien spaceship, and I feel like their queen. I want to try everything. They also ask us over and over again if we are hungry, or thirsty, or if we want to sleep; we receive so much attention that I think the only thing I'm missing is the crown. But it's all right that I don't have it because I still feel very important, with or without it.

I end up eating so much that I fall into a food coma, and they still keep bringing plates! I am given a surprise box with tons of letters in pretty and colorful wrappers inside. So many girls have wished me for the awesome trip, congratulating me on earning it, and telling me that they love me very much. Since the letters are written in English, my mommy helps me to read them all.

"Who are these girls, mamita? I don't know them," I ask her.

"They are girls who know how lucky you are to go on this trip, and simply wanted to share their joy with you."

Then, four flight attendants approach us, carrying a huge cake with candles lit, and start singing the birthday song.

"Happy birthday, Katerina!" they sing in unison.

"Wow! That's so nice!" I tell them, but then I whisper to my mommy in Russian, "Mommy, today is not my birthday!"

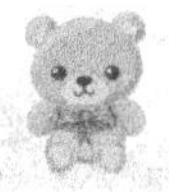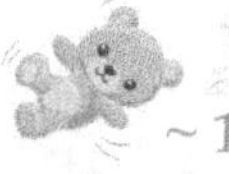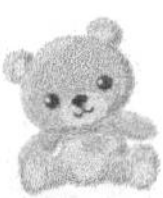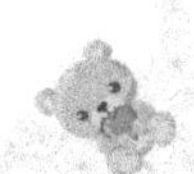

"Not yet, but soon baby, and they won't see you that day."

"Now that's just great! This is how I always want to fly."

There's food everywhere, but I have no more room in my tummy. It feels like it's about to explode! If they'd offered the cake in a box with wheels, we would surely have taken it with us, so I could eat it later. Now, I can't even look at it, much less have a bite… it's so sad, I love cakes! Next time, I'll bring a box to store all the yummy snacks they give me.

The trip is actually pretty long. Maybe it's because of the water, isn't it? Whenever I fall asleep and wake up, we're still flying. Mamita tells us that we'll be flying for some more time because of the six-hour time difference from New York.

"What does all that time difference mean?" I ask her, so she shows me her watch, turns the arrows, and then puts it back on her wrist. I guess that's it.

We're finally landing! Mommy tells us that we're going to spend a few hours at the New York airport waiting for the next flight; plus, since we are on another continent, we have to do another round of passport control, check-in, luggage inspection, and I don't know what else. Anyways, we exit the plane first, as usual, and as soon as the doors open, we hear loud screaming.

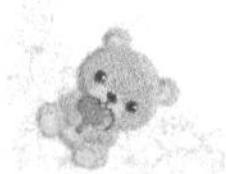
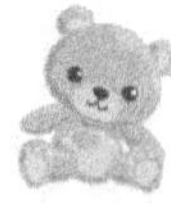
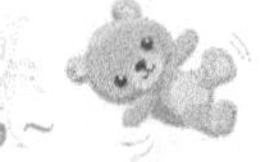
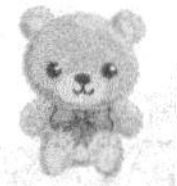

"Hooray! Hooray! Welcome, Katerina and family! Welcome!"

"Mamita! Mamita, who are they? Who are these people?" I ask her.

"They are other friends of yours Katerina, look how many you have!"

"All of them? Are they my friends? Really!?"

"That's right, dóchenka, look how much they love you."

'I didn't have many friends back in Barcelona, but everything has changed during this trip, and I love it,' I think to myself.

A few ladies welcome us and I notice they're wearing the same yellow shirts that has "Maagic Flight" words written in lilac, just like us. We're all super happy this moment, and I get even excited when one of the women hands me a bunch of balloons floating in the air. Now I have both my hands full – one with Oso, and the other with the tiny ropes that hold my new gift. However, not holding onto my mommy's hand makes me a bit nervous. I don't want to let her go, so I decide to leave my teddy under Pavel's care, but he puts it inside his backpack, crushing it.

"Watch out, Pavel, you're hurting him!"

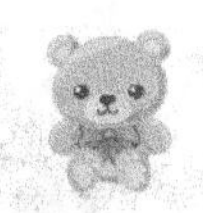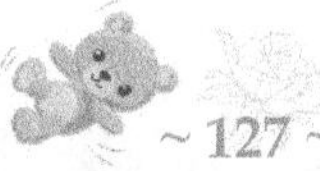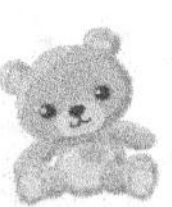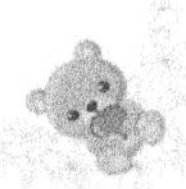

"Calm down, Katerina, your teddy bear is sleeping, he doesn't feel anything when he sleeps. See, he doesn't say anything. Don't worry, he will be comfortable in my backpack."

I can't talk much to my brother because these ladies keep asking me thousands of questions. At least now I have mamita's hand… and the balloons, which I like a lot. I know Oso won't be angry with me. He knows that I'll be right here, just a bit busy since I'm famous and I have many friends to talk with. Being famous is not so easy, you know? I mean, greeting several people, answering questions every now and then – those are kind of difficult tasks. It's feels very nice though.

We wait in the VIP room, again; there is food everywhere, with fruits, juices, cookies, donuts, anything you want! I honestly want to try everything, and I know my brothers and my mom feel the same too, but we're not hungry. Our bellies are about to explode. I don't want that at all.

Mami tells me the director of American Airlines will be arriving shortly. A lady brings me a gift bag, and a very, very nice teddy. That means Oso has a little brother now, so when I'm at school or with my family, he won't be alone. We are going to be a bigger family!

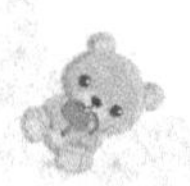 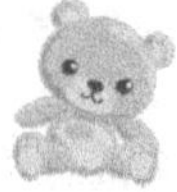 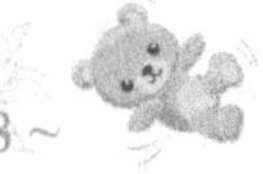 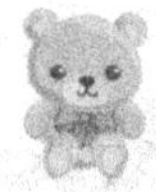

The lady sits me on her lap and talks to me tenderly, almost like my granny. She asks me thousands of questions, and there are some photographers taking pictures of us; then my family and I leave the room, and we are accompanied to the waiting area for our last plane to Orlando. I'm already exhausted from all the flights, but I'm glad to know that we will be in Florida soon.

Here in America, there's a lot of people who speak Spanish – only, their accent is slightly different – like the ladies who are accompanying us. They talk to me in Spanish, and even though I can understand them perfectly, they sound weird, like their mouths are full. My mommy explains that they are not from Spain, but from Latin countries, and I don't really know where that is. It does feel nice to have the possibility of being understood by some people on this side of the planet.

As we get closer to the waiting area, we start hearing even more screams, whistles, and applauses.

"Katerina, Katerina!"

Oh! It's for me. I'm getting used to it; the crowds, the cameras, and photographers, everything that comes with being popular.

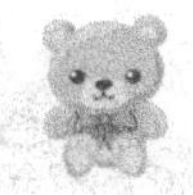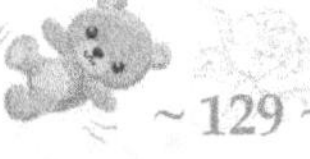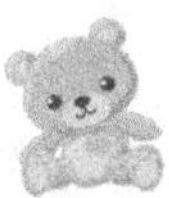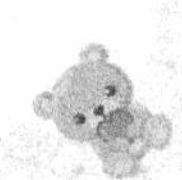

Three foreign families greet us by waving to us, and I don't know why, but I suddenly feel like crying. I turn my head towards my mommy, bury my face in her skirt and cry a river. She cries too, then hugs me tight. My brothers don't cry because they are men, and they are supposed to be brave. Men don't cry like little girls, or at least, I think so.

The families ask us about the trip and as mamita talks to them, I keep my face hidden in her skirt. I still don't know what I'm crying about. A man comes up to us after I calm down, brings me a backpack, along with another card that has money to spend at the parks. Now I have two of them!

Then the staff offers us my most favorite meals of all time! How do they know? I'm sure it was Lourdes who informed them. I remember she had asked me, back in her office, and here are tons of it! Enough to feed thousands. There's spaghetti with cheese and different types of tomato sauces, the best chocolates on earth, the yummiest ice cream, and OH MY GOD! Chocolate cake! It's like a dream. The other kids who are traveling with me also have heaps of their favorite dishes, and we can taste and eat everything. It's like a party! I eat so much my tummy starts to hurt again, but I can't put my favorite food aside. So we take some food with us to the plane, to see if I feel like eating later.

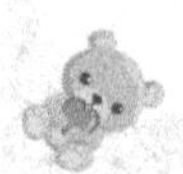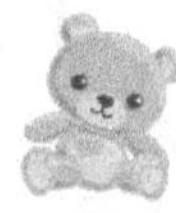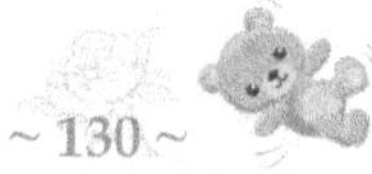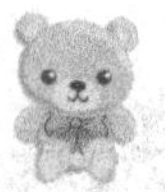

My mommy gets a blue handkerchief and I get new shoes, but the size is too small. In the end, they bring me some beautiful socks, soft like a stuffed animal, so I can continue my journey without feeling cold. It feels much better than going barefoot, and I don't stumble!

We finally get to board the plane! We cross an archway of colorful balloons and it feels like we're walking through a tunnel. This last flight ended quickly. After the plane lands, we start getting ready to leave.

As we leave the plane, we hear many voices chanting, "Welcome to Orlando".

"Oh, my dear God! Do they really know me here too, mamita?" I ask her as I'm about to cry, again. I look up to see that she is also speechless with teary eyes.

There's shouting, musical instruments, whistles, people dressed in many bright colors… it seems that we are at a party. It feels so exciting that I think my heart will leap out of my chest! I don't know what to do or what to say. I simply have a huge smile, while we walk down the long hall, joyfully.

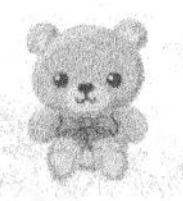 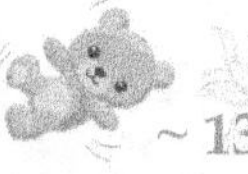 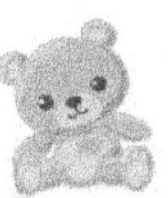 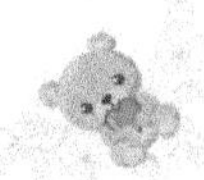

As we leave the noisy "celebrity" hallway, we approach two ladies holding a huge sign with my name, and "Welcome" written in English. They congratulate us on completing our long trip; we follow them to the spot where someone would be picking us up in a mini-bus to take us to the final point: The Magic Village.

I imagine my mommy, Pavel and Klim are just as tired as I am, but we don't complain. We take a seat with our mountain of suitcases next to us, for a bit of rest. Finally, the bus comes to pick us up. I fall asleep on the way, but my mommy wakes me up as soon as we approach the entrance of the enchanted town.

"Here we are! Hooray! We've arrived at the magic village for magic kids like me!"

Even though it's very dark by the time we arrive, we can see that the street is very pretty. There's also a sign with the letters "Give Kids the World" at the entrance, with Major Clayton, the bunny, waiting with his arms open to welcome us.

They give us a special key to our little house. It's a card with my name and our stay dates. My new friends also give us tickets to all the parks, and huge round badges with the VIP sign, so we can enter any attraction without waiting at the long lines, and take all the pictures we want… especially with my favorite princesses.

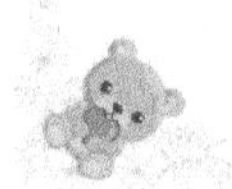 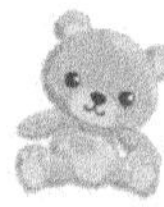 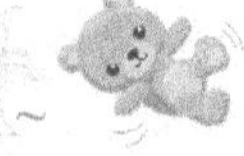 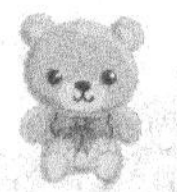

"This house is yours during your stay, and your family are your guests, Katerina," they tell me after driving me there in a toy car with all our bags.

"Wooow! It has your name! It says 'Katerina'. Look! Look!" Klim shouts.

"Where?" I ask, excited.

"Here, Katerina! Look! In front of the house!"

"Oh, yes! I see it! It's true!"

In front of the house number 188, we see Major Clayton holding a "Welcome Home Katerina" sign.

"How is it possible, mommy?" we ask her, all at once.

"This trip has been specially prepared for Katerina. Everyone here knows who she is, even Mayor Clayton! He was waiting for you all this time."

"Wow!"

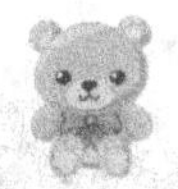 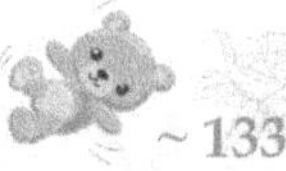 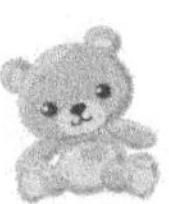 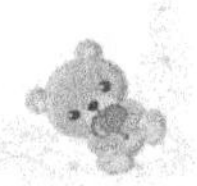

It would be hard to get lost, or even enter the wrong house. The man who drove us there in the toy car, drops us off, and we start investigating the entire house; it looks magical because of how beautiful it is; there are two big rooms, a huge bathroom and an even bigger living room with a kitchen. I can't believe it's mine.

"I am going to be sleeping with mommy!" I shout at my brothers so they wouldn't get ahead of me, but they don't even listen to what I say. Pavel and Klim are enthusiastically running all over the place. They find out that we can set the Jacuzzi mode in the tub, with foam and bubbles.

Mami tells us to take a shower because it's been a long trip and we probably picked up a bunch of germs along the way. She says the beds are really clean, so my brothers start filling the bathtub with foam; but when I go in, there's foam all the way up to the ceiling. Ugh! It's chaotic! I quickly give Pavel and Klim a look of alarm and we start screaming for mommy to help us. She gets a bit mad at us, but we immediately clean up the mess. Phew! Once we finish, mommy fills the tub carefully, and lets us play with the foam. I love it! This is so much fun! I can hide inside it, just like with the clouds, which I sadly couldn't taste.

We finally get some time alone, with nobody shouting, or giving us food, and I feel sleepy already. In my opinion, it feels like we flew for thousands of weeks, without a normal bed.

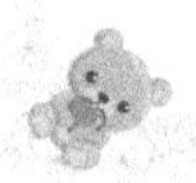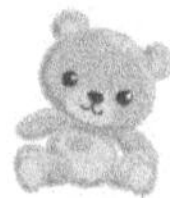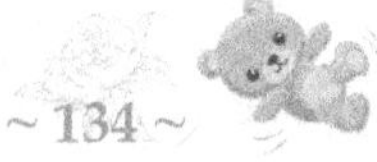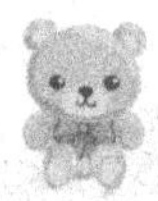

The princesses are all hidden. I need to be strong and regain my energy from the whole trip to get to know them. That night, I dream about laying on some soft white clouds, while Rapunzel and Tiana play with cloud balls by throwing them to each other, like it's snow.

THE MAGIC BEGINS

I hear some delightfully cheerful music in the background when my mommy wakes us up.

"Dóchenka, Pavel, Klim sinochki, come on, get out of bed. It's time to have breakfast and get to the parks."

The moment I hear "the parks", my sleepiness disappears. We jump out of bed to take a shower, brush our teeth, get dressed, and leave my little house to visit my favorite princesses.

We are starving already, and there's tons of different meals at the restaurant where we have breakfast. They've prepared omelets similar to the Spanish', but when you bite into it, it has cheese that stretches for miles away. It's delicious! The pancakes are the best though; they are fluffy like cushions. I have never seen anything like it. The ones my mommy makes are thin.

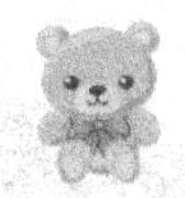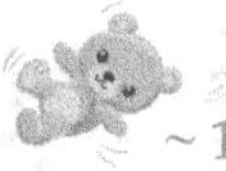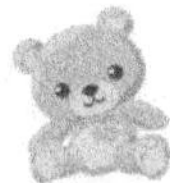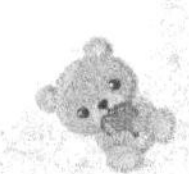

Here, they also put some syrup on top, with whipped cream and berries. But since I don't like fruits, I ask for mine without it.

Oh! And the chefs can be seen by everyone as they cook, isn't it fun?

Once we finish, we go to take a look around the Magical Village. There's so many tiny houses that seem like fairy houses. At some point, a tree suddenly starts talking to us, which causes us to jump back in fear, but then we laugh out loud; his name is "The Miraculous Tree", and not only does he know how to talk, but also to fulfil wishes.

And guess what? There's more food! We walk by a pizzeria where you can order any kind of pizza you want, but we can't even think about it right now. An ice cream shop around the corner serves the biggest gelato in the world and everything is free! None of us – my mom, brothers, and I – want any more food for now, even though it looks yummy, so we leave it for later.

The yellow bus, that will be taking us to the first park, is waiting for us. We need to hurry so it doesn't leave us behind. After we get in, I realize that this one is huge, and there are a lot of children with their moms and dads; it feels like we're lifelong friends. The bus finally starts moving and I'm super happy knowing I am about to visit the authentic princesses' houses.

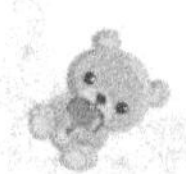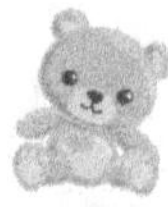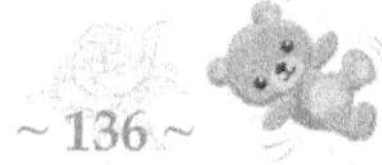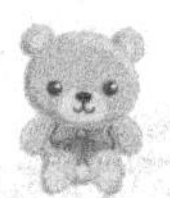

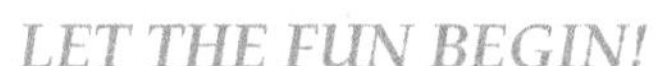

LET THE FUN BEGIN!

We are in the Magic Kingdom! The streets are huge, with a massive number of cars, expansive roads, and palm trees that reach the sky. They are so tall that you can barely see the top, and the heat is just too much. It seems that summers here are much more intense than those in Spain or Ireland. Here, the heat is blistering.

"Here it is! We're here, mommy!!! Look at the sign, Katerina!" my brothers scream with excitement when they see the "Magic Kingdom" sign.

I already want to jump out of the bus, but we have to wait for our stop. Those are the rules. Once we can finally get out, we can go inside the park without waiting in line at the entrance because we have the magic badge they gave us at the Make-A-Wish office.

"Look! Mommy, look! Those are their houses! Here it is mommy!" I scream with joy when I see the palaces of the princesses at the distance.

"It's true, honey."

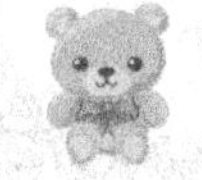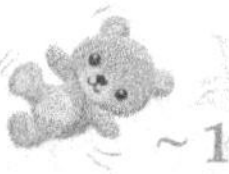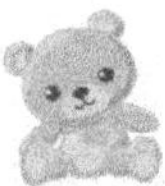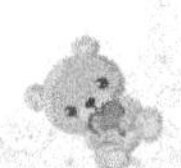

At the entrance, we meet Minnie and Mickey Mouse who give me a strong hug, and I think they might know who I am too... or maybe it's because of my badge. We take pictures with them and dance together. My mommy bought us a notebook so Klim, Pavel and I can have their signatures forever.

As we continue, I realize that there are many attractions. For God's sake! They're enormous! I don't want to leave until I've tried out every single on. Suddenly, we see a long line that stretches for thousands of kilometers. What could it be that's so interesting? Surely we were all connected because our feet led us there at the same time.

"It's her! It's her, mommy, it's her!"

"Who, dóchenka?"

"It's Rapunzel, mommy, there she is! Come on, quickly, come on! She's waiting for me. Come on!"

We arrive at a special entrance where there wasn't even a single person in line. I am eager to rush inside and get to know Rapunzel. The real Rapunzel.

A lady comes to us and asks, "Make-A-Wish?"

"Yes!" we respond impatiently and cheerfully.

"Wait a second."

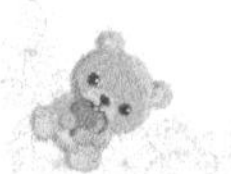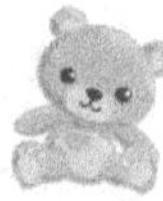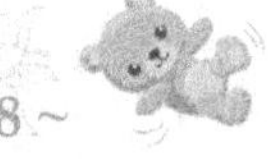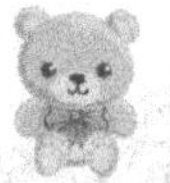

The lady goes to the other line, closes it, and gives us access to where the princess awaited. I'm not dreaming! I'm really going to meet her! For real! I run towards Rapunzel. She stretches her arms out to reach me, and I can't help crying when we finally hug each other. I feel like she is my best friend, you know?

"What is your name, sweetheart?" she asks me when I calm down a bit.

"Katerina."

"Hello, Katerina! What a sweet name you have. I am Rapunzel. How old are you, my little angel?"

"I am eight years old."

"Oh! You are a big princess. Where are you from, honey?"

"I am from Spain..." Then I think for a bit longer and continue, "...and from Ireland too." Honestly, I am a little lost about where I am from.

Luckily, she asks me easy questions and I feel like we understand each other perfectly. She is so beautiful! Her long, lilac dress is sparkly, her blonde hair is braided... that's what I love most about Rapunzel. When I grow up, my hair will look just like hers. I feel so happy! I came to visit her in her castle! It's a dream come true. We take thousands of pictures together, and even though I want to stay for hours, there are other kids waiting to see the princess, so we must leave.

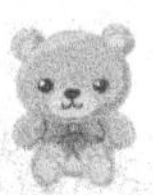 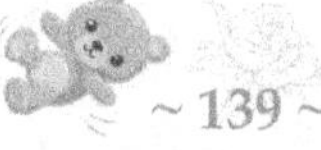 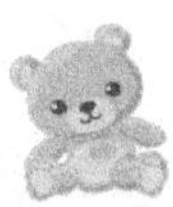 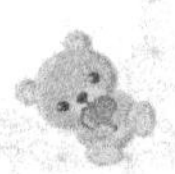

Almost immediately, we go to meet Tiana, who is with her prince. He is no longer a frog, which means that the spell has been broken! How nice! They are both lovely! Once again, we pass through without queuing. Now that's cool. Tiana is my other favorite princess, and of course, I want to take as many pictures of us as possible, so I can look at them every day. They will be in my memory forever. It seems to me that Pavel is in love with her because he wants to take pictures of just the two of them. He even made her prince jealous by asking him to step aside a bit. Everything is so magical! The princesses have been waiting for me all this time, and now I am with them in a fairy tale.

Now let's have some fun! I don't care how many rides there are, we're going to try them all. First, we come across a broad elevator, which goes up really fast, stops mid-air for a few seconds, and suddenly opens the window to throw us out. It's a good thing we're strapped securely to our seats, and also have a metal bar to hold on to. Phew! That was really fun, but scary at the same time! We spend the day at the park, trying out all the rides one by one. And when we got tired of walking so much, we took a break in the VIP area, which has air conditioning, comfy chairs and sofas to rest.

It takes us an entire week to visit each park. The first one we go to is Magic Kingdom, the second is Epcot, and the third one is Universal Studios.

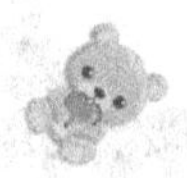
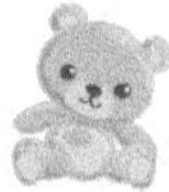
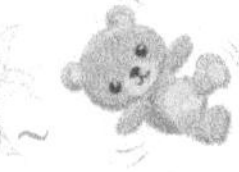
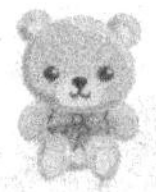

They're so big that we had to walk nonstop during the third and fourth day to explore them. Some of the rides are really cool, so we take several turns riding them, and on our last tour, we get to caress the dolphins at SeaWorld. We also take a tour though the Harry Potter village, with its snow-covered roofs, and hundreds of characters with whom I was able to talk and share some of my secrets.

One time, a man approached my mom after noticing that we went everywhere without waiting in line.

"Are your children superstars?" he asked.

"Yes, actually, they are," she told him, and then we rushed off to try out some other spots.

One day, we wanted to stay at the Give Kids the World village, without going to any of the parks. There's a number of attractions there too, with activities of all kinds, and a huge pool that looks like the beach. I love swimming, so I don't have any problem staying in the water the whole time. The town also hosted a barbecue, with tons of food, different flavors ice cream, and blue or pink cotton candy.

Another afternoon, we decide to simply rest in my little house, eating pizza and ice cream towers that we can't even finish. In my mind, I dive into it and savor every last bite, but my belly tells me to stop, and so I do. Let's avoid another food coma.

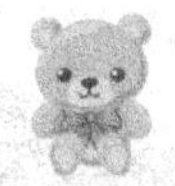 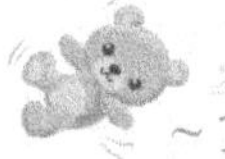 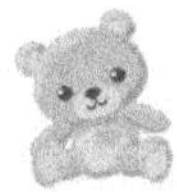 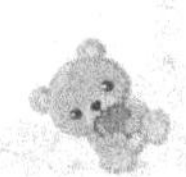

Our end of the day return home is full of expectation because we know that when we return from the parks, there will be gifts laid out on the table for us. On the bus ride home, we repeatedly discuss amongst ourselves about the surprises that awaited us.

All the way through.

Major Clayton bunny comes to visit us with his wife, Mrs. Marry, to say good night, with hugs and kisses included. They are really nice. We take pictures together, and they look hilarious with their huge heads. Then Mrs. Marry takes me to bed and leaves a basket with chocolates and stuffed animals, some in Clayton's likeness, but wearing glasses.

On the last day of our vacation in the magic world, the people of the kingdom throw a Christmas party, and Santa brings many gifts for all the children. I choose a giant Barbie doll with two different wigs; my brothers pick some board games. The whole town sings and dances joyfully, and although it is rare for me to celebrate so many things at once, I find it really emotional.

You see, in this place, every Saturday is Christmas because some children are very sick. My mommy told me that some of them don't really get to experience these holidays.

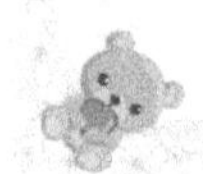 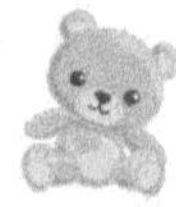 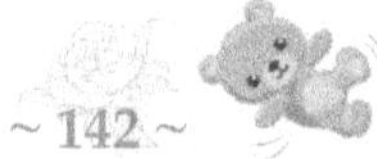 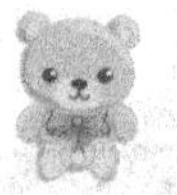

THE RETURN TO TARRAGONA

I received so many gifts that they almost don't fit inside the suitcases, but it turns out my mom knows some spells too and manages to make everything fit. On the last day of the trip, we eat our pancake breakfast with syrup and whipped cream. All the visitors bid the staff a tearful goodbye, who give us colorful necklaces as a parting gift; plus, they give me a bright star with my name on it, and a diploma of graduation in magical parks. I knew it! I am a magical girl!

"Goodbye, Magic Village! Thank you! I had a wonderful time at your mysterious places of princesses and wizards. I will never forget them! Oh, and of course the talking tree...I wish I could take you home with me!!!"

The trip from Orlando's airport to New York's went by pretty fast; they recognize us and offer mamita a flight that will take us straight to Barcelona, so we will be home much sooner.

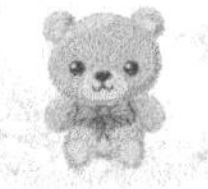
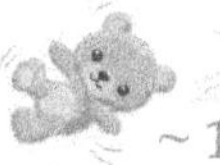
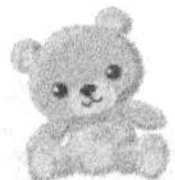
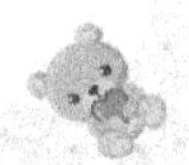

When we finally arrive, my daddy is waiting for us. But... what a misfortune! My pink suitcase, which is very important because it contains all the presents, got stranded in New York. Only that one! I feel like crying, but mommy tells me that it will be delivered tomorrow, or the day after. I don't even notice when we got home because tiredness and sleep won me over. The best thing is that the very next day, my daddy brings me my suitcase with everything safe inside, thank God!

We celebrate my birthday in Tarragona with the whole family. Wow! I'm already nine years old! I'm going to wear a beautiful turquoise dress with yellow straps, that Minnie gave me. It has her face printed on it, and so that I can feel like I'm still in her world.

Everyone gives me lots of presents, and mamita prepares a delicious meal to eat together before singing the birthday song like we always do, and then we eat a chocolate cake, my favorite. It was a nice day.

We spend it by telling the family about our magical journey to the other side of the world, beyond the seven seas and seven oceans, where humans can only visit once in a lifetime..

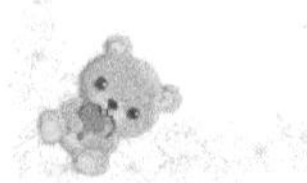
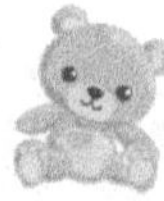
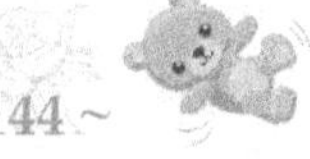
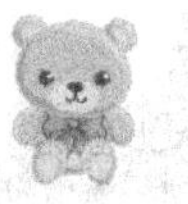

THE RAIN AWAITS US

We wake up early to get to the airport in Reus, near babulia's place. We will be returning to our house in Ireland, so this will be the last flight of all our adventures... for now. Wow! In fact, it's the seventh one in just two weeks. I'm already an expert, not only as a passenger, but also as a pilot. Mami, Klim, Pavel and I get to the plane that will take us to Charlestown's Knock Airport. It takes us about two hours to arrive. This flight is faster than the others, and much faster than going by car, or by boat. It is wonderful to be able to go everywhere in a flash! I'm not saying I didn't like the other trips; just that the plane is like a rocket.

The rain welcomes us as soon as we land in the city. That's our new home. Olga, mommy's friend, comes to pick us up, and in the blink of an eye, we are home.

The weather in Ireland is very different from Orlando's, where we were roasting. Here we have no choice but to wear lots of clothes to avoid getting cold. Mamita turns on the heating quickly and we have to wait a while for the house to warm up. In the meantime, my brothers light up the fireplace, and we start unpacking.

I love my new bears and dolls! I can't wait to introduce them to their family.

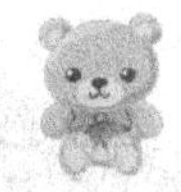 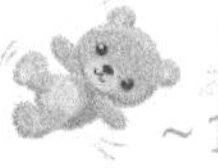 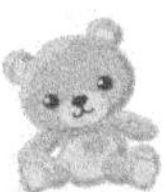 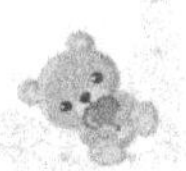

It is not so easy to keep the house warm, you know? Mami has to ask a truck driver to bring "Kerosine", a liquid that makes it happen. Then he fills up a huge tank outside that can't ever be empty, or we would freeze.

NEW LIFE IN CHARLESTOWN

I like everything about Charlestown: our house, the school, the people... everything. The folks are very pale, unlike the people in Spain, where almost everyone is tan because of the sun. Maybe that's it! The sun is to blame! I mean, here it hides all the time and that might be the reason people don't get tanned.

I can't help remembering how incredible it was to visit the Magic Kingdom and its princesses. The teachers at school get angry with me because I don't pay too much attention to them, but I don't care. I don't really understand much of what they say, for now.

As time goes by, I start to understand English a little better, and can even manage short conversations with my classmates, who are very patient with me. Thank God! I also got to know some of the kids here. We don't need to talk to communicate because it seems that we understand each other much better by playing together.

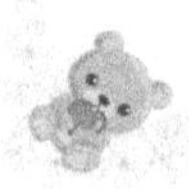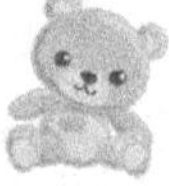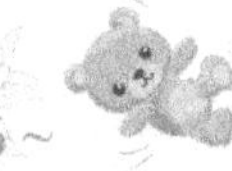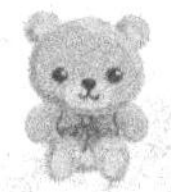

My best friends are Charles, who is originally from China, and Victoria, whose family is from England. After school, we play in the park and have a lot of fun; there is a pyramid made out of ropes that I have difficulty climbing, since I am afraid of falling. My friends give me a hand, encouraging me to make my way to the top. It makes me very happy. Getting back down is nicer since there is a curved slide that I love to ride. That's actually the reason I try so hard, despite the wobbly ropes. It's worth the effort! Charles, Victoria and I compete to see who can go down the slide the fastest, or who can do it first.

It rains a lot in Charlestown, so we can't go out that often. Instead, we get together at someone's house, and turn it upside down. Our parents don't get angry because they make us pick up everything after we finish.

Charles' house is gigantic. On the first floor, his parents have a Chinese restaurant, and whenever we go to visit him, they give us something nice to eat; his actual house is on the second floor where they have many toys, posters, paintings, carpets, dolls… everything in a Chinese style. Charles' parents are good people. They let us spend hours and hours playing – the bad thing is that sometimes we forget to do our homework.

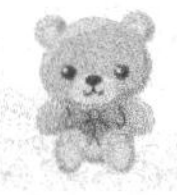
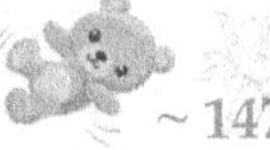
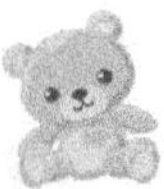
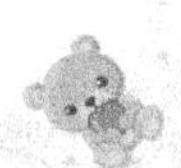

My friend Victoria's house is inside the forest, a little further away from the city; it has trees around a huge muddy field, and lots of beautiful animals of all kinds. I didn't know you could have so many at home. There are horses, cows, sheep and guinea pigs, which I didn't like, at first, because they reminded me of rats, though they're bigger with straight hair. But the truth is, they are super quiet and don't bite. Her family also has two dogs, plus five or six cats... it's a good thing there's enough space.

Victoria's favorite pet is a guinea pig that she named Princess. She loves her so much that they even sleep together! I've had some trouble with it before, but then I begged my mommy every day to let me have one. I didn't succeed though. Anyway, this animal is really smart. She understands English whenever we play with her like a doll; Victoria and I bathe her, feed her, dress her up in cute clothes and she obeys us for everything. She doesn't run away like the cats and never gets angry. Cats are another story... they always flee or pull out their claws. That's the main reason I prefer not to play with them.

Sue, Victoria's mom, is very loving towards me. Sometimes when we have sleepovers at their house, we playact scaring each other with the flashlight under the blanket, fooling around all night long, while her parents are resting. Sue never gets mad at us – not even when we can't wake up in the morning. She always brings us breakfast in bed with a nice smile.

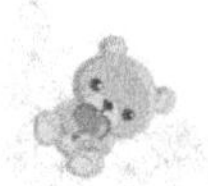 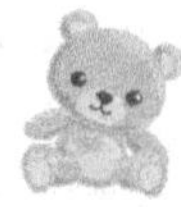 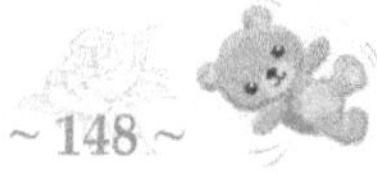 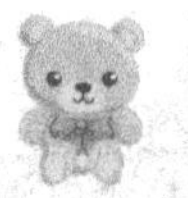

"Girls, what would you like me to prepare for breakfast?" she asks in English, of course, because nobody speaks Spanish in this country.

"Pancakes!" we answer together.

They taste so good that we even end up licking our fingers. She pours maple syrup and whipped cream on them. Yummy! We feel like princesses... or more like queens, because the princess is Victoria's guinea pig.

Sometimes after leaving her house, we go back to mine and continue playing while our moms talk in the kitchen, enjoying some tea and cookies.

In short, I have my first two friends: Charles, and Victoria, whose mom, Sue, is also my mommy's friend. Olga, a Russian lady who has her own beauty salon called VIP, is also another friend of mommy's. Sometimes she styles my hair and gives my brothers a haircut whenever they need one. Mamita's friends are very nice people!.

THE IRISH EXPERIENCE

Time has definitely flown by. We were supposed to be back in Spain by now, but my mommy says we're going to stay here for another year.

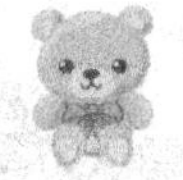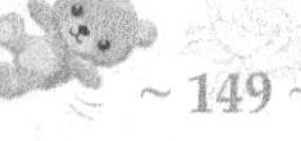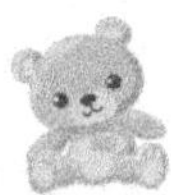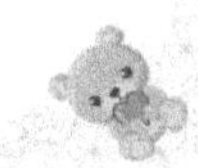

That's fine by me since I find Ireland to be a very nice country. Besides, it would be sad to leave my new friends behind. However, Pavel doesn't like the idea and always gets irritated whenever mommy mentions it. As for Klim, he says he doesn't care either.

The decision has been made. During the summer vacations, we will be flying to Spain to have some real fun. There, we can hang out with the family and go to the beach as many times as we want – until the new school year begins. Both Christmas and Easter holidays follow the same routine. That is how it will be for a while.

My brother's school is right next to mine. I wanted to be with them, like in Spain, but I still have two years of primary left. During my fifth year, Mr. Brian McDermott, the principal of the school, will be handling our classes. The classrooms always have two different groups, while ours will be grouped with the sixth class. As the months passed, I started to like Mr. McDermott, even though I'd been terrified of him at the beginning of the year; to be honest, he ended up being the best teacher in the world. I love my Irish school life! We are like a close-knit family where we all love each other.

I also learned to speak English well, and can even correct mamita when she says something wrong. Over the years, we've met so many wonderful people, learned about their cultures and all the things they were passionate about.

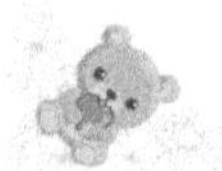
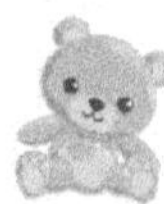
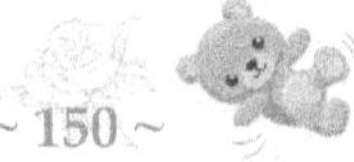
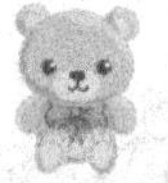

Every six to eight months, I have to go for my medical check-ups at the children's hospital in Dublin. Since the results have been positive so far, there is nothing to worry about. Both the doctors in Ireland and Spain are relaxed, and so are we.

It's a great experience visiting Dublin with my mommy because I don't have to go to school afterwards. Also, on the way to the hospital, we always stop for gas and breakfast at a station called the Green Apple, which has a coffee shop with delicious meals. On those days, we leave the house so early that it's still dark outside. So mommy lets me sleep a bit longer in the back seat, with a warm blanket and a soft pillow.

Mamita loves croissants, but my favorite food from that place is hashbrowns – a plate of grated potatoes made like crunchy croquettes. It's either that, or a chocolate muffin with hot cocoa. Our Lady's Children's Hospital is quite close to the coffee shop, so I don't go back to sleep once we leave because mami drives us there super-fast.

The city of Dublin is a bit sunny, at least, more than where we live. It even resembles Barcelona. My doctor there is excellent, although, sometimes he makes us wait for about three hours in the waiting room; nowadays, we've gotten so used to carrying something that might entertain us during that period of time.

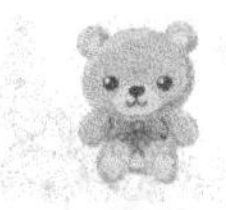 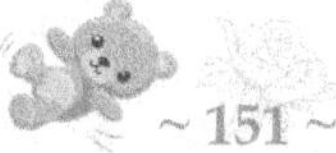 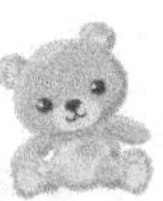 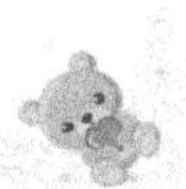

When we leave the hospital, we always stay in the city for a while to do some shopping downtown, or walk around O'Connell street, which is really nice. There are bars, restaurants, markets and stores. So mommy and I have fun, like we're on vacation, even if it's only for one day it's very cool! When we get back home in the evening, we spend the whole way talking about anything and everything, unless I fall asleep in the back seat.

STRANGE SUSPICIONS

We have lived in Ireland for almost three years now. Mamita says that we won't be moving back to Spain yet because she would have to find a new job and a new home. That would be a bit complicated, so for the time being, this is our home. Also, as stated by her, it's better for Klim to finish his two years of high school left before college.

I'm ten years old now and being the big girl that I am, I've already begun to understand adults' conversations much better. The sixth class has been a great experience, and the best part is getting to join Klim in secondary school after I graduate in half a year. Mommy, Klim and I like it here, and we are used to the city.

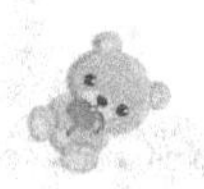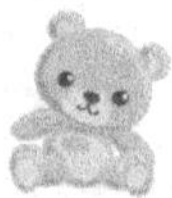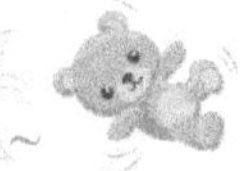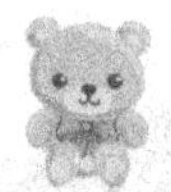

Nevertheless, Pavel is in his last year, and has been studying hard to pass the exams for the university that he wants to go to in the USA; although he's been accepted to Trinity College in Dublin, he is determined to find a scholarship outside Europe. Pavel tells us not to worry because he would call every day, but I don't want him to leave us since I will miss him a lot.

It's true that Charlestown, as small as it is, doesn't have many fun places to hang out, there are bigger cities like Castlebar or Sligo nearby which have movie theaters, bowling alleys and lots of stores of all kinds. During our stay in Ireland, we have visited many gorgeous places like Cork, Galway, old castles, waterfalls and mountains. In other cases, whenever my granny yaya, Liubasha with my cousins, and my uncle Ilusha come to visit us, we'd take them to all of our favorite places. Like the famous Titanic museum in Belfast, where people don't use euros, but the England's currency called "pound".

After the surgery and the chemotherapy, my tumor seemed to have shrunk since it had been poisoned by the treatments. It didn't have the strength to continue growing and then fell asleep. It hasn't disappeared completely, however, which is the reason why we've examined my head with MRIs from time to time.

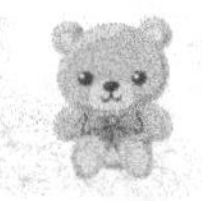
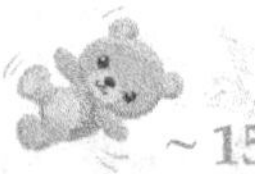
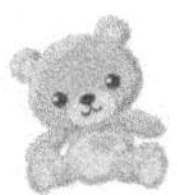
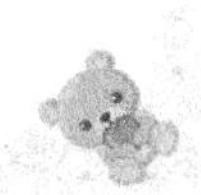

We are currently at the Dublin hospital with Dr. Kapra, who looks a bit worried; he usually talks to me very slowly, so that I can understand everything. He always asks me about school, the trips to Spain, my friends, my favorite subjects and teachers, or whatever. It's a normal day like any other, we don't expect bad news...

"From the MRIs, I've observed a slight growth of the tumor," Dr. Kapra explains while looking at the results. He pauses and continues right away.

"I don't want you to be scared, it could be just a mistake. It's possible that the results here don't coincide with those in Spain because they are not the same machines."

The last MRI images had been taken in Spain during the summer vacations. We always try to repeat them in Barcelona and then bring them back to him; maybe he wasn't so scared because these MRI results are from a different machine.

"We have two options..." he continues talking. "We could repeat the images here, in a month, or repeat them in Barcelona with the same machine that made the previous images, to compare them."

"We'd better go to Spain to repeat the scan there as soon as possible, we can't wait a month."

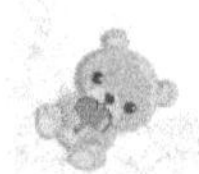 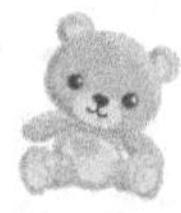 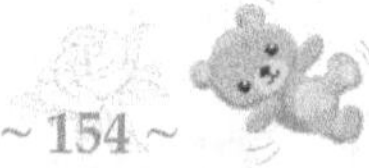 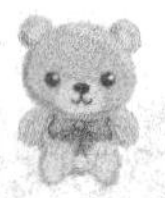

To be honest, I am terrified. The last thing I want is to go through those ugly treatments that made me lose my hair, again. When we left the doctor's office, my mom said, "Don't worry dochenka, everything will be fine. We've never done MRIs here before, so it's probably a mistake. Here the machines are older than in Spain... so we'll travel there to make sure everything is in the same place."

That calms me down, so I stop thinking about the false alarm to concentrate on the fabulous day we are going to spend in Dublin. I'm already daydreaming about eating something tasty somewhere on O'Connell Street, like we always do, walking around the stores, or the Chinese market, and at the end of the day, going to IKEA to buy something for our house. It feels like there's always something missing around our home. Anyway, I love being alone with my mommy because we have a great time laughing at her jokes and talking about anything.

We return home at nightfall and, on the way, pass by the LIDL, ALDI or TESCO supermarkets to buy some food for the whole family. I always carry a change of pajamas and a blanket, in case I get sleepy. Then, I only have to change clothes and move to the backseat. It's much more comfortable that way because when we arrive home, I can go straight to bed, without even brushing my teeth. It's quite a festivity for me.

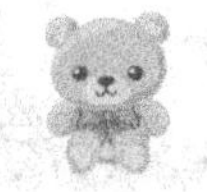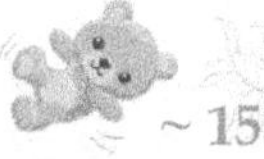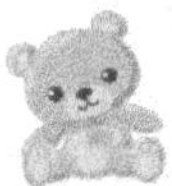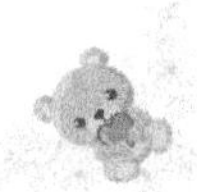

Mamita wakes me up in her sweet voice when we get home, and if I don't want to get out, she says, "Do you want to stay the night in the car?"

Obviously, I don't. It's cold there. Although it's not easy for me, I get out of the car, dragging my feet, fall into bed and fall asleep right away. Then mamita helps me take off my shoes and covers me with a blanket.

TRIP TO SPAIN

Spain, here we go! I'll get to see babulia and daddy! Even though it's not a vacation trip, I am really excited. The most important thing is that my family will be there. Woohoo! This time, mamita can't go with me, so her friend Andres will be coming to pick me up and take me to Barcelona's airport where daddy will be waiting for me.

Once we arrive at the Vall d'Hebron hospital, we have to wait for my turn, as always. The MRI waiting area is pretty boring. There are not many toys, and the few left have missing pieces. Besides, the place is lonely. I don't like it, at all. It isn't like the oncology section where you have so many things to play with, and the volunteers make up fun games for all the children. I even have some friends there; some of them are the same ones who come by every treatment day, while some others are from the summer camps that AFANOC (a Hospital's organization) hosts, which I've attended several times.

It's finally my turn! I don't like being alone in the MRI room, so daddy always comes in and stays with me.

Since the doctors want to look deep inside my head, they take the images using contrast – a kind of liquid that lights up my body parts so they can be seen better. Earlier, they used to inject it into my arm, but now, they injected it into my chest, right where I have the port-a-cath; I needed that weird coin for the chemotherapy, or the blood tests, so they didn't have to prick my veins every single time. It isn't really necessary now, but the doctors still haven't removed it. Anyway, my parents usually put a special lotion that mamita keeps in the fridge, so that the shot doesn't hurt. I really hate that part; whenever the liquid passes from the needle to the port-a-cath, I feel something cold spread through my body. It feels disgusting!

I can watch a movie while the machine is running, but it is very loud, like a construction zone. I've tried to talk loudly over the noise, but I can't even hear myself. The doctors hand me earphones to concentrate on the film, but I still can't hear it. It's annoying. Luckily, I fall asleep most of the time, and one of them asks me "Are you actually going to watch the movie or just count sheep?" a bunch of times, making everyone laugh, including me.

The moment the images are finished, we go to doctor Sabado's office in the oncology section. He is a good friend of my daddy's, who always likes to make jokes about calling him "Domingo".

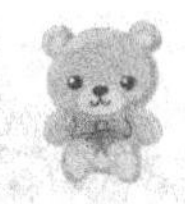
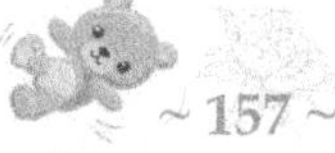
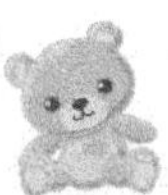
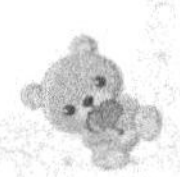

Whenever those two get together, the conversations and giggles are endless. After leaving the hospital daddy gives me a chocolate and a pink cocoa donut for snacking. My favorites!

I'll be staying in Spain only for a few days this time. The best thing about it is getting to spend some time with babulia, and better yet, she will be travelling with me to Ireland and stay with us there for a whole week.

Once the new MRIs have been compared with the last ones from Ireland, daddy gets a CD that contains the results and gives it to me in a packet. It's really important that my mommy gets it safe and sound. I am responsible for that, so I have to take good care of it. I don't worry because it's control exams, you know, just to make sure everything's fine. Plus, those are adult things and I know trust me with the delivery because I've proved they can count on me.

BACK TO IRELAND

I love Spain but I have to return to Ireland with my granny. Since this is an unplanned trip and the summer holidays haven't begun yet, I know I will have piles of homework to do, as soon as I return.

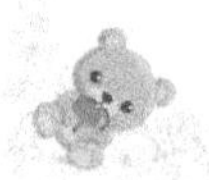
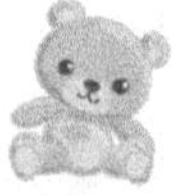
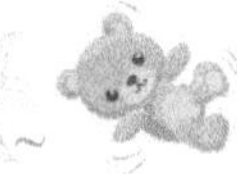
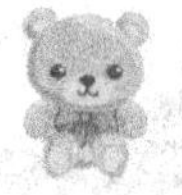

A whole week of missing school, to be precise. Nevertheless, mamita will help me. She knows how to recap the classes and explain them to me in a short time. She's brilliant! When I have kids, I want to be like her. Moms are like encyclopedias. I only have one, but I think they are all the same.

My daddy drives babulia and me to Barcelona's airport where we'll be taking a plane to Dublin. There are no more direct flights, like when we flew from Charlestown to Reus, and the other way around. Once in the city, we have to go to nearest the bus stop which is right at the exit, and take the bus home without making any transfers. My granny doesn't speak English, so I have to be on watch to make sure she doesn't get lost. It is my duty, which means that I have two responsibilities now: both her and the confidential documents that daddy gave me. Believe me, it's not easy.

The bus ride to Charlestown is quite long and lasts for almost four hours. If you wanted to go to the bathroom, you have to hold on until the driver makes a stop in Longford; he says "No special stops are made, for anyone", not even for the kids. That's the reason why I got used to peeing before the trip. Plus, leaving the bus scares me because my mommy told me that one time she had gone to the bathroom and they hadn't waited for her. And that they'd left with all of her bags! The stop had lasted only five minutes, instead of ten! She was able resolve it anyway, but had almost missed her flight.

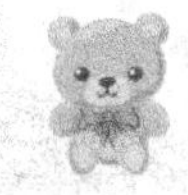 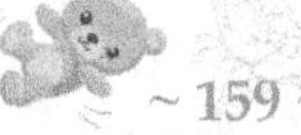 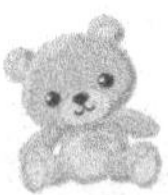 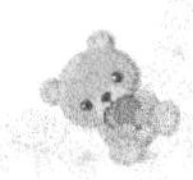

Since my mommy told me about that experience, the Longford stop scares me into being extra careful. So if she's not with me, I'd rather hang on; besides, this time, I am responsible for taking babulia home. It's better not to take my eyes off her or she might get lost.

I'm afraid I might pee my pants; maybe I could tell the driver three times that I'm going to the bathroom and run back fast in a minute… but what if he leaves? Gosh. If mami were here, she would tell him to wait for me, but my granny doesn't speak English and it's not the same.

My granny is so focused on each bus stop and they all sound the same to her. She's scared of going beyond our city. So I have to keep asking the driver over and over if we have arrived at Charlestown yet. As soon as we approach Charlestown, you can already see the difference from Spain: it's raining cats and dogs.

We get out of the bus and walk home for about ten minutes. I made it! I was able to bring both my granny and the CD perfectly! Uff... what a big responsibility.

My brothers are very happy because we've finally arrived, and even more so because our babulia will be staying with us for a week

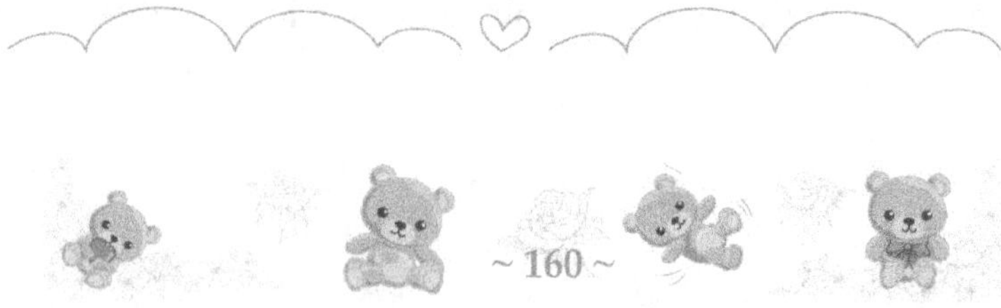

THE WORST NEWS EVER!

A few days later, my mom talks to me about something I wish I hadn't heard...

"Honey, do you remember that your trip to Spain was because the MRIs from Dublin didn't match the ones from Barcelona?" I listen carefully without suspecting anything wrong, and she goes on.

"Well... ummh... it turns out that there is no mistake, baby. It seems that the tumor is growing."

Hearing that made me remember everything I had to go through a few years ago – the hideous haircut, the painful surgery, the hunger, the thirst, the lack of energy, the nausea and the headaches. Even the worry for my whole family. I suddenly feel sad and scared. I don't want to have that stupid tumor. I wish it would go away from my life. Forever!

"Why, Mommy?"

"The doctors said it woke up. But don't worry, my little princess, they are not giving you chemo. There's another much shorter treatment. We already have the images that we are going to deliver to Dr. Kapra, and he will surely offer us Radiotherapy, which only takes ten minutes a day, for about two months. The specialists even want to start the treatment in summer.

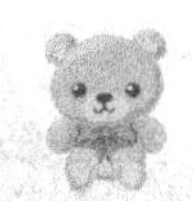
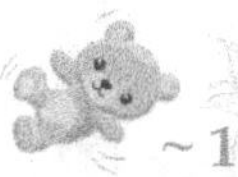
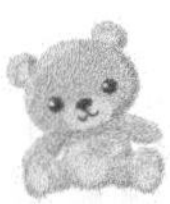
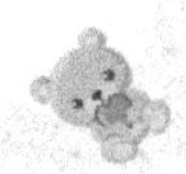

That's perfect, right? I mean, there's no school during July and August, so by the time you go back no one will notice. What do you think?"

I'm speechless... What other options do I really have? The news sounded horrible at first, but as my mommy explains more and more, I notice that it isn't too bad; although, it's sad that I won't be able to go to summer camp like I usually do every year. I really wanted to see my oncology friends. There's one where we're allowed to bring our siblings, so I always invite Pavel and Klim, and we have a great time for a whole week. The best part is that there are no exams – just fun, fun, and more fun. Who doesn't love that? Every summer, I look forward to those camps.

One of them is named AFANOC and the other is named AECC. The latter usually takes place in a hotel in Salardú named Val de Arán, which is in the mountains. Sometimes they even organize winter gatherings for skiing in Andorra, it's amazing! I really enjoy attending them, and I feel like my happiness will be taken away this summer – all because of the horrible news mommy just gave me.

"Maybe I can go to at least one of the camps, right, mamita? My friends will be waiting for me. I've been connecting with them all year long. Now what, mamita? I really want to go!" I plead with her.

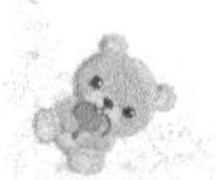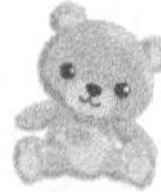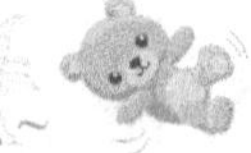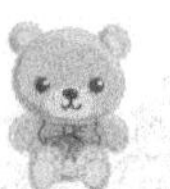

"I'm very sorry, sweetie, I know how much you'd like to go, but you can't this year. It is important to do the treatment. We will surely go next year..." she pauses, and then tries to comfort me. "Radiotherapy won't be too bad. It's not like chemo. This time, we won't have to spend the night at the hospital. It will only be about ten minutes a day and that's it."

I keep a poker face because I know I'm about to cry, so my mommy immediately hugs me and says, "Everything is going to be okay, baby. Now the most important thing is your health, then we will have time to enjoy all the camps you want. You'll see. Ok dóchenka?"

"Ok," I answer begrudgingly.

A few days later, mami drives us early in the morning to Dr. Kapra's office in Dublin. The routine is the same as always: we arrive, wait for our turn, he calls us in, then asks me about school or my trip to Spain, they both throw in some jokes, and finally he comments on the results.

"I've seen all the MRIs from Barcelona and those do match with ours. I'm very sorry. We must do the radiotherapy treatment."

"Is there any other alternative?" my mommy asks him.

"Well... not really. Not right now. This is all we can do."

"We were offered the same treatment in Spain..."

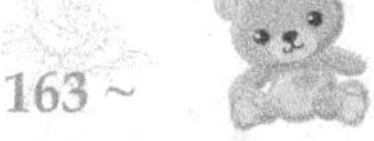

"You don't have to go back there. We can give you housing during treatment here in Dublin."

That sounds great to me. Living in this city for a couple of months might be nice; but my mommy looks worried. She asks Dr. Kapra lots of questions and breaks down in tears. Did he say something bad? Probably... you know how it is, if I see mommy crying, I follow.

After we leave the doctor's office, my mommy is calmer and says, "Don't worry. Everything will be fine, little princess. We can stay either here or go to the Xuklis house, which we already are familiar with... we like it, we really like it, right?"

She stays silent for a few seconds before replying, "Besides, we will have our family close by."

"The Xuklis House?" My eyes open wide. I don't think about it much more. "Yes! I do want to go there."

The first time I'd gone there, there was an opening party and I had a great time with all of my AFANOC friends. Another time, my daddy and I had stayed there for a couple of days. That house is beautiful; it has a huge garden, spacious rooms, and it's full of nice people. This time we could stay for two whole months, in summer! Wow! Just imagining it makes me really happy.

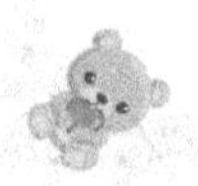 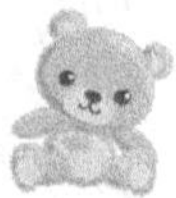 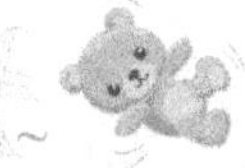 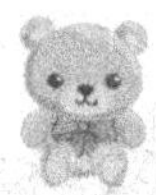

"All right, dóchenka, then that's what we will do," my mommy continues. "As the treatments will be from Monday to Friday, that same day, we could travel to babulia's house in Tarragona to spend the weekends with the family. Then we would return on Sunday night to Barcelona. Or perhaps at dawn on Monday."

"How cool! Then I want to go to Spain!" I love the idea of being with babulia and my uncle Ilusha.

"You'll see, baby, we're going to have a great summer after all."

It's February, 2014. My mommy is busy organizing our trip to Spain, while the boys and I continue our studies. Pavel has his head down while preparing for the SATs. He will be taking the test in Dublin, which will determine if he's going to study in the U.S.A.; it sincerely upsets me. It's not fair that he wants to go so far away from us. My mom is also helping him with the paperwork for his trip to the other side of the planet.

This trip to Spain will be similar to the one we made when we first arrived here – only, in the opposite direction. It will start by car, then by ship, and finally by car again... it's going to be a long journey. We better start getting ready from now. Mamita says we have to take the car out of the country because we can't register it in Ireland and, plus, it needs to be checked. I don't understand much of this, I just know that's the reason we'll be travelling by car and blah blah blah. Children don't worry about that kind of thing; adults do. If it has to be done, it has to be done.

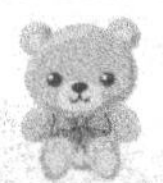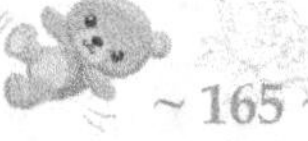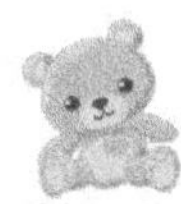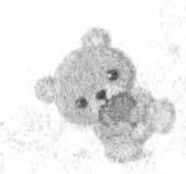

WHAT'S WRONG WITH ME?

Since the tumor has grown again, my fingers suddenly start getting numb and my head begins to hurt. I feel horrible. As soon as my mom notices that, she quickly takes me to Castlebar's Hospital in Mayo County, which is pretty close to home. There, they do another series of emergency MRIs.

"Wow! What a long medical record you have, Katerina!" they say. "Compared to the images you brought, there's no growth. You don't need to worry."

They give me some pills so that I can feel my fingers again and that's it... But a few days later, I start getting dizzy, and don't just see double, but triple. And similar to how it was before the chemotherapy, I can't see things clearly. It's weird. I don't like it.

"If it gets worse, you will have to receive treatment sooner," the doctors tell us.

Accelerating the treatment means doing it in Ireland, which I didn't want. I want it to be in Spain, with the awesome plans my mommy made, but there are still a couple of months left for this school year to end.

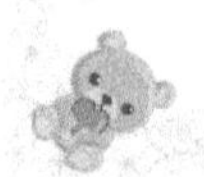
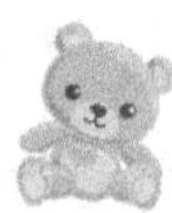
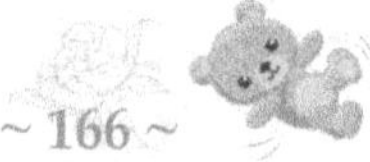
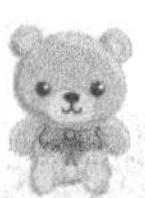

During the remaining months, I have to take some medication to feel better, but they don't work. Even though the pain is awful, I hold on for as long as I can so that my mommy doesn't take me to get radiotherapy in Dublin. She has already organized a fun trip to Spain on the ferry for us. I want to go there.

The last day of school is here. I don't feel very well during my "primary graduation", but still manage to participate in our recital. I'm feeling calm because all of the teachers know about my health. I know they will keep an eye on me, just in case anything happens. We'll be hosting a concert for the parents where the class usually sings something nice, and everyone stands and applauds.

In the middle of the event, I suddenly feel very dizzy, losing notion of where I'm standing. My vision starts to blur and everything goes dark. I feel like I'm falling, slowly. Luckily, the wall is right next to me, so I lean against it before sliding into a chair. Mommy notices it immediately and runs towards me, helping me to sit, while Mr. McDermott opens all the windows. I don't think anyone else saw me because they'd acted quickly. My breathing returns to normal by the end of the song, so I can rejoin my classmates.

KEEP DRIVING!

Summer vacations are finally here.

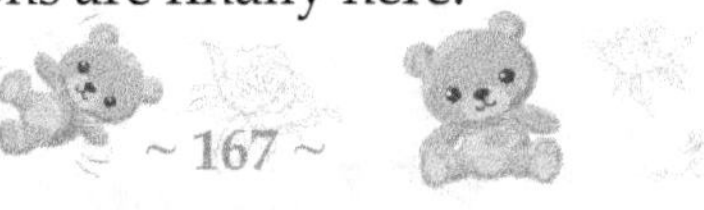

On one hand, I feel excited because I'm going to see my family, but on the other, I'm scared about the treatment that awaits me. What will it be like? My mom frequently keeps asking me about how I feel and says she will do her best to get to Spain as soon as possible. I know she is very worried. This time, mami won't make any stops in France, not even one. Although, in case of an emergency, she will look for the nearest airport. I hope nothing happens because I don't want to be away from my mommy and my brothers. I need to stay strong. Whatever it takes. Mamita needs my help since it's not easy to organize everything by herself. The best thing I can do is be a good girl. If I take the pills the doctors gave me for pain, everything will be fine and she won't have to worry so much.

The day we're set to leave in June finally arrives. We pack our bags and put them in the car with all the gifts we've bought for the family, before getting in and driving off to Spain. Just like when we came to Ireland. As we travel along the same road, I forget about my body ache since the excitement about the trip blankets everything. I am so happy!

Pavel has grown so much that he is already learning to drive, and he is constantly asking mami to let him take the wheel. On this trip, he is supposed to help her with the driving, so she can rest.

"Mamita, let me drive! You need to save energy. The road is long!"

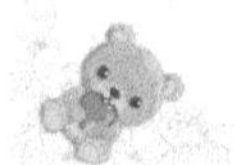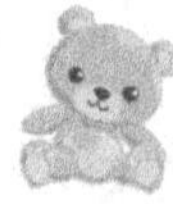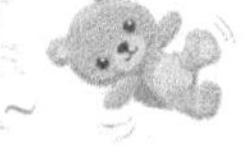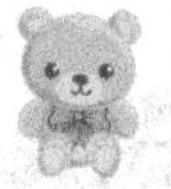

My brother knows how to drive very well. He's sixteen and old enough to take the theory test, but he has to wait one more year to get his actual license. We almost have a heart attack at a police checkpoint, because we nearly got stopped with Pavel driving. Phew. It's a relief that he looks older than his age; the cops made a sign for us to move on. We got lucky!

We finally arrive at Rosslare's port. I almost forgot how fun boat trips could be and the routine is the same: we board, sleep in the mini-cabin, and lastly, get to Cherbourg's port in France. Or as Klim says, "We moor".

Everyone keeps asking me how I feel every five minutes, or if I need anything... I tell them I'm fine, even if it's not true. It's a little white lie. The thing is that I want to be with my brothers and my mommy. I don't want to be sent on another transport to Spain.

Mommy, the boys, and I have a very long journey across France. We sleep in the car, eat in the car and only make small stops to stretch our feet, fill the gas, and go to the bathroom; otherwise my mommy drives, drives, and keeps driving... poor thing, I would like to help her. I'll do it once I'm Pavel's age and learn how to drive.

This road seems endless, so my brothers and I ask her over and over again, "When will we get home? How much longer?"

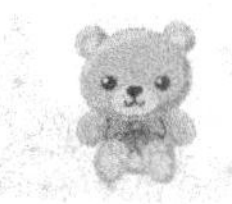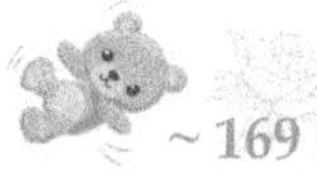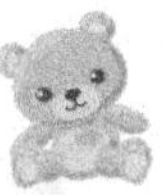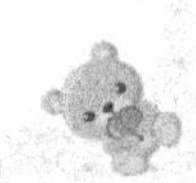

"There's still a few miles left," Mommy answers, and constantly tells us which town we are in. We have a GPS that marks how much time we have left before we get home.

During the nights when we sleep, she still keeps driving and driving... How is it possible?

"We are almost in Spain, kids," she says finally.

Finally!!! Our beloved Spain!!! Even the weather seems to change instantly, just by putting one foot on its side… or as people say "when the rubber hits the Spanish road".

It's really weird that borders can't be seen. We know where they are because mommy informs us. Plus, the phones go PLIN! PLIN! PLIN! with new messages. When that happens, it's because we have already crossed borders. Hurray!

We stop at a McDonald's in Figueras city. Phew! It feels good to take a break and eat something warm. Mommy takes advantage of the moment to call everyone and let them know that we will be home in about two or three hours. When we arrive at Tarragona, everyone is waiting for us. Babulia, Ilusha and my daddy help take our stuff out of the car, hugging us tightly. I feel very happy to be here!

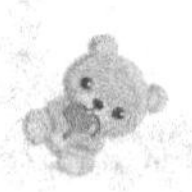
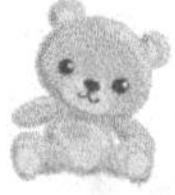
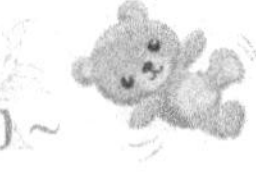
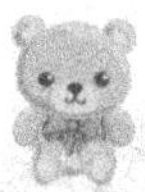

I think mommy has superpowers because she managed to drive without stopping for even a second. As soon as we arrive, she disappears, locking herself in my granny's room to get some sleep – she must be exhausted. We'd better be quiet so she can regain some energy..

RADIOTHERAPY

It's time to move into the Xuklis house in Barcelona. The room that's assigned to us is huge, with two double beds and a big sofa; there is enough space for everyone to get comfy. We can even invite babulia or my daddy to stay with us! There's also a fridge to store our food, a TV, a desk, a big balcony that connects to the garden, where mamita can dry our laundry, and a bathroom with a shower… all to ourselves.

In the common area, there is a kitchen with a huge table in the middle, and includes many stoves and ovens around. There are large shelves, for families who stay here, to store the nonperishable food, some more smaller refrigerators, and many, many utensils. Sometimes the gardeners leave delicious fruits and vegetables on the table, and everything comes straight from the garden!

In the Xuklis house, there is also a playroom, and another huge dining area where we can all eat together. The people who stay here are usually very united. It's like a huge family.

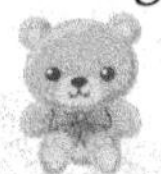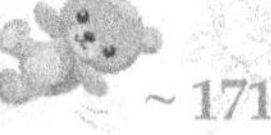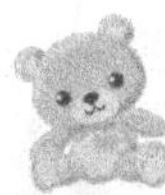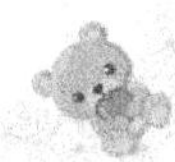

Klim rides the subway with us, every morning, to a computing school. Pavel decided to stay in Tarragona because he wanted to spend his last vacations in Spain with his friends, yaya, his father and Ilusha, whom he considers to be his brother; besides, he has to complete some formalities at Madrid's U.S. Embassy for a student visa.

It's time to go to the Hospital and start our summer routine. We wake up early on the first day. The nurses take my blood sample, as usual. Then we visit the radiation oncologists, who lead us to an odd place, hidden through many doors and hallways. They explain to me that I will have to lie totally still during the treatment, since it uses a laser beam pointed at my head. To make sure I won't move during the treatment they will be making a kind of mask for me, but I don't really understand. How is it going to work? The doctors dip a cloth full of holes in hot water, stretch it all over my face, and then wait a few seconds for it to get solid.

"Are you ready, Katerina?" they ask.

"Yes, ready."

Actually, it's the opposite, but I can't say much because I have to wear that thing... whether I like it to or not. Besides, I want to show both the doctors and my mom that I'm brave, and that there's nothing to worry about.

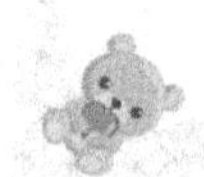 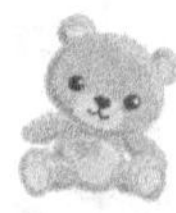 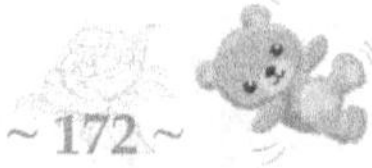 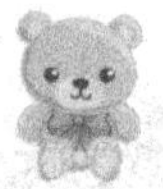

They inform us that the treatment will commence tomorrow, and that I will have to remain alone in the room. This time, mamita can't come inside with me. Everyone will be watching me through the monitoring cameras. Scary! This is like a prison.

RADIOTHERAPY BEGINS

We eat our favorite breakfast: croissants. Mommy likes them with condensed milk and a cup of hot green tea, while Klim and I enjoy it with chocolate and a cocoa milkshake – his being strawberry pink, and mine is chocolate brown. Yummy! Sometimes I add more powder than I'm supposed to and it makes my milkshake sweeter and a lot more chocolatey, but shhh!!! Let's keep that between us.

Once we finish eating, my brother goes to school, and I go with mamita to the Vall d'Hebron Hospital, which is right next to the Xuklis house; barely a ten-minute walk away. As soon as we arrive, I started to remember the chemo days because they took the same tests. However, what follows after receiving the results is totally new and gets super strange – it feels like we are in a thriller movie.

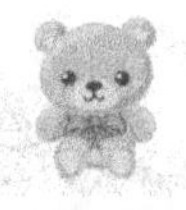
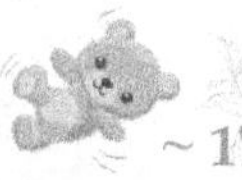
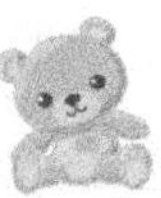
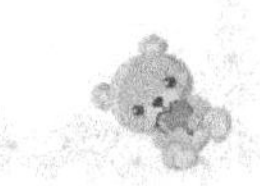

Someone comes to guide us to a restricted zone where the doors open using a special key, that only people who work at the hospital have. That's weird. What if mamita and I want to escape? We would be doomed. We walk through many corridors until we finally reach another waiting room. Ugh. There isn't a single window... the place is creepy. Seems like a basement. There are a couple of people waiting for their turn, and I think that the treatments may not be as short as the doctors had described.

A nurse takes me to the room where I'm going to have the treatment. I immediately feel like we could be friends. She is so cheerful and kind to me; even though it's a short way there, her jokes make me feel comfy. So much so that I almost forget that my mommy has to stay outside.

The room is as cold as the North Pole. I've never been there, but I know it must be this icy. There is only a giant machine in the room, and the special table where they'd taken my face measurements. Everything is fine, until the lady puts the mask on my face, before attaching it to the table. I CAN'T BREATHE! What if something happens? How will I get out of here? The only thing that calms my panic attack is thinking about mamita. I know she won't leave me, so I take a deep breath and close my eyes. I want this to end quickly.

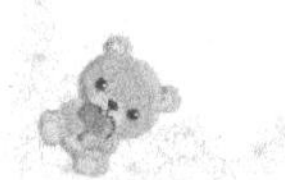 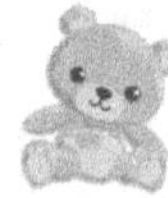 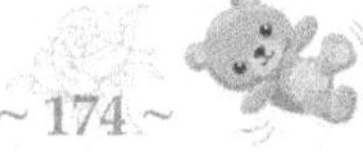 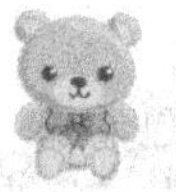

'It will only take ten minutes, I have to be strong!' I whisper to myself, while hearing the nurse's footsteps move away.

I am left completely alone, with my face tacked to the table.

The robot starts moving, as if it were alive, holding its arm behind me and to the right side of my head. It stays that way for a few seconds before passing to the other side and repeating the process. That weird thing keeps doing the same over and over again... I guess that's called radiation.

It's uncomfortable being held in this room. They said it would only take a little while, but it's been hours... I can't stand having this disgusting mask on my face one more minute; it feels like I'm drowning, it's too tight, and itchy. Maybe the doctors took the wrong measures. I clench my fists tight to hold back my tears. I'm a big, strong, brave girl. I can do it! Plus, my birthday is coming up soon, and eleven year old women don't throw tantrums like little babies.

Suddenly, the nurse comes in, and congratulates me on getting through my first day, and for my good behavior. Then she takes off the awful mask and accompanies me to the waiting room. Everything will be fine; now I can breathe much better.

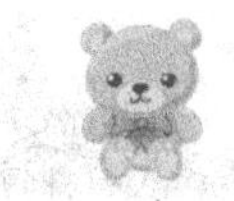 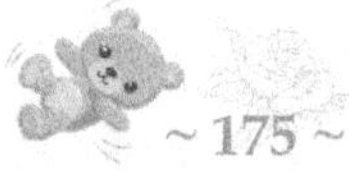 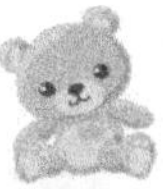 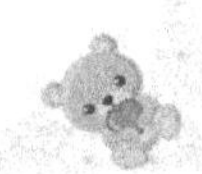

"How did it go, dóchenka, how did you feel?" my mommy asks me, hugging me tightly and filling my face with kisses.

"Good, mamita, but I could barely breathe, the mask is tight and smells like garbage, I don't like it."

"I can imagine, baby, but that's the way it has to be so there's no movement of any kind. They can't allow mistakes in this treatment, honey… the radiation has to be done with precision."

"I can hold on, mommy," I answer, sighing.

One less day. Moving on from despair, I feel good.

From Monday to Friday, it's always the same mundane routine, unless the test results are not good. In that case, the session gets cancelled until the next day. Some afternoons, we wait for Klim to return from computing school so we can go to a friend's pool since the Xuklis house doesn't have one. That's how our life went by during the two months of summer vacation. I wanted to see my friends at the Val d'Aran camps, but my mom tells me not to worry because I will be able to go next year. At least we can do whatever we want once we leave the hospital, and also spend the weekends in Tarragona. I love spending time with my family. I forget about the treatment and feel that summer vacations are real.

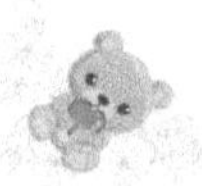 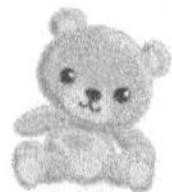 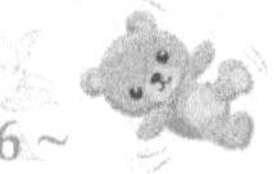 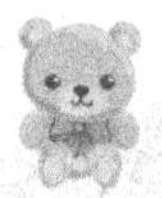

During the second week of the radiotherapy, I start feeling a bit weak. I don't know what's wrong with me; just that my body feels weird. One night, I leave the room, go to the kitchen and walk around the huge table twice, then eat some cherry tomatoes and return to my room. I'm really surprised when I woke up, "How did I get here?" I think to myself. Our mini-cabin's door is closed using a key I don't have. So if no one opens the door, I would have to sleep on the couch outside. In that moment, I decide to ring the room's doorbell.

Mommy opens it and asks me, "What are you doing here, Katerina?"

"I don't know," I answer, confused.

The next morning, the oncologist explains that I was "sleepwalking", which was caused by the medications I've been taking. I tell Klim about everything that happened, and we laugh out loud.

"It's okay, Katerina. Good thing you didn't go outside, because you might have stumbled upon a wild boar from the nearby mountain; and even better that we are not on the second floor... you could have gone out on the balcony, walking along the edge of the railing. Can you imagine? Scary!" we giggle.

"That's true! Good thing nothing like that happened." And we keep on laughing together.

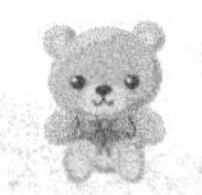 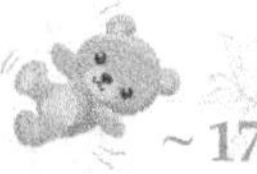 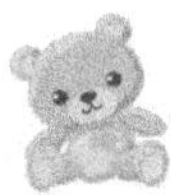 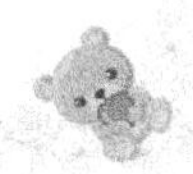

Mamita is looking for activities to distract us during the day, like going to the movies and eating the colored popcorn that we love, going out to parks, visiting friends. Sometimes there are moments when I don't feel like going anywhere so we stay at the Xuklis house, where volunteers organize some activities for everyone. And if I feel sick, I can always go back to my room to get some rest. Radiotherapy makes my face swell up; even the mask they made feels tighter each day. It occurred to me that the doctors could make bigger breathing holes for my nose, so that I can breathe easier, but they don't. I guess I'll have to hold on.

TWINS' BIRTHDAY

It's my mommy and Liubasha's birthday! Since my cousin Adelina's birthday was yesterday, the family will be celebrating all three birthdays on the same day.

We eat at a nice hotel restaurant and have fun at the swimming pool, and even though, I feel tired I keep going; I truly want mamita to enjoy her birthday to the fullest. The party is for the twins' and yet they give us a surprise after dinner: there is a pink disco-bus waiting for us outside. WOW! I've never seen anything like it; it has colorful lights, loud music and drinks – no alcohol, of course. It's a dance hall, but with wheels. Awesome!

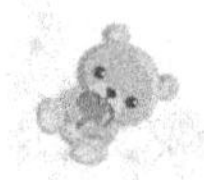
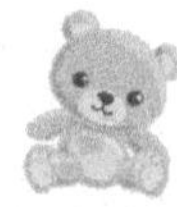
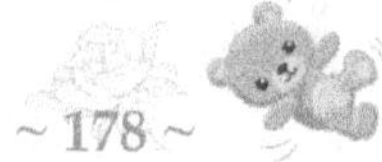
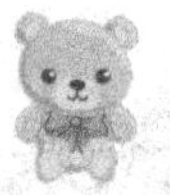

All of us dance so much that the bus moves side to side. I hope it doesn't fall over. After driving all over Barcelona, we are exhausted from all the singing, shouting and fooling around. The driver takes us back to the restaurant and bids goodbye. The parking lot was actually a good spot for a quick photoshoot with the flowers that were given to my mommy, Liubasha, and Adelina. So before we leave, we stay there for a while. Everyone starts posing, except for the boys who tell us "those are girly things".

At the end of the day, it's time for our guests to return to Tarragona, except Adelina, who will be spending the night with us at the Xuklis house. In the morning, mamita and I will take her to the station where she will board a train to Madrid. She lives there, and also trains with a national rhythmic gymnastics team. It was a wonderful day. I'm happy – a bit sore, but very happy.

We're only a few meters away from Xuklis house when the car suddenly stops. What happened? It seems it doesn't start back up, so my mommy sends us home alone while she waits for the tow truck. You would think that with Adelina, Klim, and I, we are a big bunch, but we're afraid of walking in the middle of the night through the dark streets; besides, there is not a single person around...

On the way, a huge wild boar suddenly appears, making us run while we scream in fright.

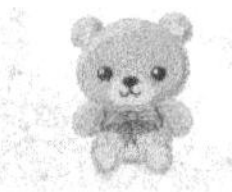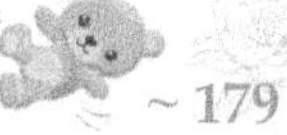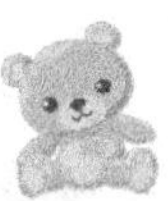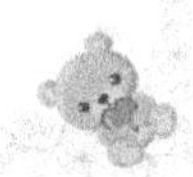

Since I was carrying the leftover cake from the party, I ran ahead of everyone because I thought the boar might smell it. I don't want him to catch me, otherwise he'll eat the cake... or me.

We reach the Xuklis house, with hearts racing. What a relief that we escaped from that animal, and that I saved the birthday cake I will eat for breakfast! It's midnight so everyone is sleeping. We better go to our room quietly. The beds seem like a paradise right now, or maybe it's the tiredness that makes us see them as such? Anyways, as soon as we touch them, we fall into a deep sleep, so much so that we don't even notice when mommy arrives.

The sun comes out and it's time to say goodbye to my cousin. Since the car broke down, we couldn't drive her to the train station, so she had to take a taxi. Adelina almost forgot her phone charger in the rush. Luckily, I saw it and ran with my mommy to give it back to her, along with a piece of fruit for the road.

We get to my cousin just in time! I didn't know it, at the time, but after that day, I wouldn't see Adelina again for many years. My life and destiny would change completely.

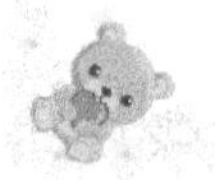
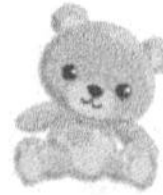
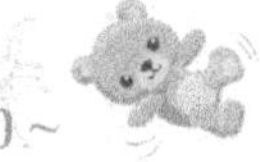
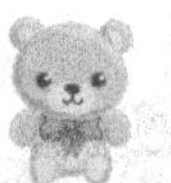

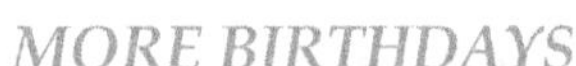

MORE BIRTHDAYS

The few weeks of treatment I've gone through makes me get tired faster – not to mention my legs, my belly, my arms, and my whole body, but especially my face, got so swollen that I look like a red, ugly balloon! It's awful. My favorite dresses barely fit me, and I don't even want to look at myself in the mirror anymore.

Although my energy is not the same as before, I'm very excited about babulia's birthday; as I'd said before, we celebrate many birthdays during the summer. The last ones were just one month ago and now it's my granny's turn. Another party! I want to give her a lovely surprise. Mamita and I prepare a Russian cake that she recently learned how to cook. It's called "Medovik" and it looks delicious. She tells me that we have to bake eight layers separately, and then spread a cream between each one; right as mami is putting the cake in the oven, I run a hand through my hair, tearing out a tuft, unintentionally.

"Mamita!" I scream with fright, showing it to her. "What is this? I don't want to be bald again, mami, I don't want to!"

I start crying in fear.

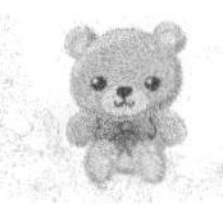
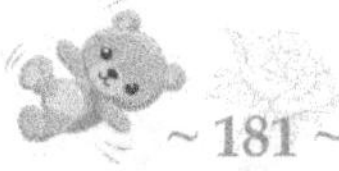
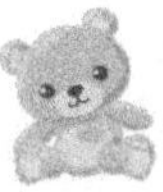
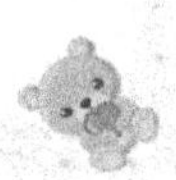

My mom runs towards me, holding me tight.

"Everything is going to be alright, little princess. Don't worry, you won't lose all of it. Besides, it's the hair in the back and you can't even see it. Soon it'll grow back more beautiful and nobody will notice. You'll see, dóchenka!" she tries to cheer me up, but it doesn't make me feel any better. Even if it's just a handful that can't be seen, that lock of hair is no longer on my head.

The other parents in the kitchen also try to calm me down. They say the sweetest things to me, but I can't stop weeping... until the cake almost burns. I forget everything else in that moment, getting lost in my thoughts while we set the Medovik's final touches. I know my hair won't grow back any time soon. I just hope the section that the treatment burned won't be so visible and the radiotherapy ends soon.

It's babulia's birthday! We arrive early and I join the family's children to help set the table, chairs, cutlery, plates and napkins. Everything has to look great. Dinner is ready, the table is well decorated, and we also wear our prettiest clothes before waiting impatiently for the many guests who would be coming. The party proceeds normally: with lots of noise, loud music, piles of presents, and at the end, the cake that my mommy and I made, decorated with lighted candles.

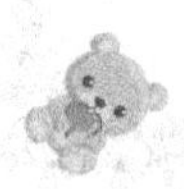 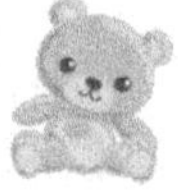 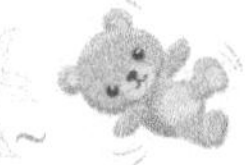 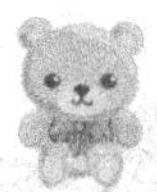

As always, we sing the birthday song in four different languages: Spanish, English, Russian and Catalan, in that order; it's very funny because just when people think we've finished, we start again, and so it takes a long time to blow out the candles. Maybe the factory should make bigger candles, so they last longer while we complete our tradition... Anyway, everybody loves the cake. They say it's yummy and ask us for the recipe. I feel very proud to have helped my mommy prepare it.

After the party, we go outside and realize there's a band playing music next to babulia's house, what a coincidence! We join the neighborhood party, as if it was just for her, and stay until the last dance.

GOODBYE FOREVER, VALL D'HEBRON HOSPITAL

We are so happy Pavel got his visa to go study in the USA in October. There is only one month left! On his side, Klim finished his computing studies and was given a nice yellow diploma with huge letters. Now I have a brother who is a university student and another one who is an expert in computers. That sounds really cool, to be honest!

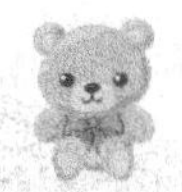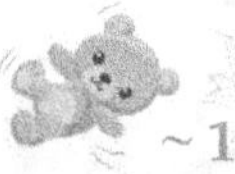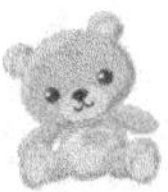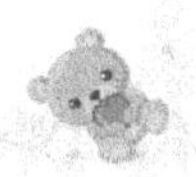

When I wake up every morning, I see a lot of hair on the pillow, and when I take a shower, more falls off. I can't even make my one or two ponytail hairstyles anymore. I'm afraid to touch it; luckily that's happening at the back of the head, so I don't have to wear wigs, head scarves or hats. Mamita always carefully makes me a loose braid in the lower half and that's enough. At least it looks nice. Good thing I only have a few more treatment sessions left. I hope time passes quickly. Within a month, we'll be going back to Ireland and I can forget about the Vall d'Hebron Hospital.

The last day of my radiotherapy has finally arrived! The last visit to the doctors, the last MRI control, and the last good-byes to all the people at Xuklis house, who made us feel like family... I think everything turned out to be just fine. We can now go home, and return to our normal life. The radiation oncologists offer me the mask as a souvenir, saying that I could paint it with pink, lilac or any colors I liked, but I don't want it! The last thing I want to remember is what it felt like to wear that hideous thing: the fear, the lack of air, the tightness, the screws, and that cold room in that basement that felt like a dungeon.

WE ARE GOING HOME

The whole family has gathered around to wish us good luck for the long journey ahead.

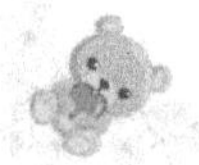
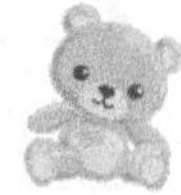
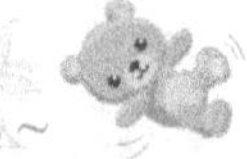
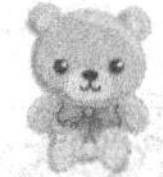

We already know the route perfectly, and mommy is an expert at making round trips. It'll be a piece of cake! I feel weak, but happy because we're going home; plus, I love traveling, and there's no need to worry even if I feel any ache since the doctors gave me ibuprofen. What a relief the tumor has died!

We only make one long stop to regain some energy during the whole night. The rest are much shorter; just enough to eat and go to the bathroom quickly. This summer seems hotter than any other. So, during one of the stops when mamita can't take it anymore, she throws a towel by the shade of a tree and takes a nap, while the boys and I play for some time. We get pretty excited once we arrive at the port. It doesn't matter that we have already travelled by ferry because it always feels like the first time... My brothers are impressed by how fast it moves, but me, I'm in love with the landscape. We are so captivated that we don't even realize that the ship has already moored at Ireland's port – our home.

School started a week ago, but mamita tells us that "it's just a small delay". Anyways, she accompanies me on my first day to let the teachers know about the radiotherapy. I just found out that we have a new principal, who is kind of a wicked witch – she yells at everyone and constantly gets angry; along with a new vice-principal who feels so self-important and ignores the students, like we are too small to be seen. I'm not surprised that nobody at school likes them.

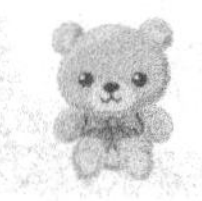
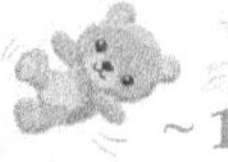
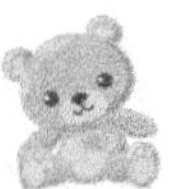
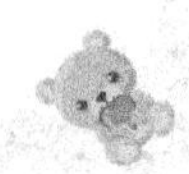

I can't believe October is here. Pável wakes me up at dawn to say goodbye, asking me to stay strong and to behave; I don't want him to leave, but I know he has become a man. So I promise him to be the best girl on earth... indeed – the universe! At that moment, I cry so much that I almost flood the room. I feel like I miss him already.

"I love you, bro," I whisper in English, hugging him tightly.

"I love you too, sis." He gives me a forehead kiss.

I watch him as he walks out of the room and I scream, "I will miss you a lot!"

"I will miss you too, cutie!"

After a few minutes, I hear the sound the car makes when it starts, and I couldn't help running to the front door to see him one last time.

"Bye, Pavel! I love you very much! Goodbye!" I cried, waving my hand.

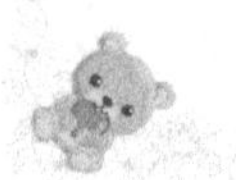 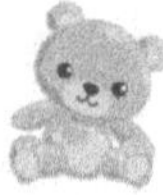 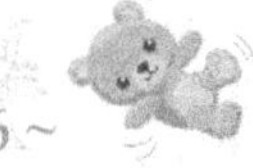 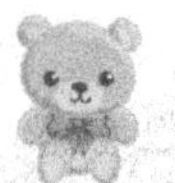

Dublin's airport is pretty far from home, so I better not keep them long. That day, Klim and I walked to school in silence. It's very strange not having our big brother with us… almost feels like are missing some body part; in spite of everything, I'm very happy to have another brother, whom I know will help me with my homework and protect me from all the bad people around. We are not alone, that's for sure.

Pavel's room will be mine from now on. He left a Mayo County's flag hanging on the wall. I remember when he found it long ago, dropped on the street. It hadn't been much important then, but now, every time I see it, I feel that my older brother is right by my side. That banner is like a lost treasure.

A few days after school started, I suddenly feeling bad. Any loud noise began to bother me, giving me such a headache that I often ask the teachers for permission to go home, and they call my mom to come and get me right away.

"I don't feel well, mommy."

"You probably didn't get a good sleep, honey. Do you want to get some rest?"

"Yes, mamita. I need to sleep."

You see, my mommy is like a magical medicine. Just being by her side or hearing her voice immediately makes me feel better.

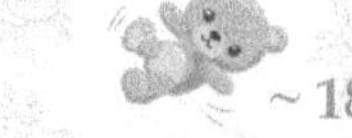
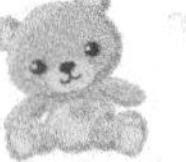

The first thing we do when we get home is eat a fresh salad and some rice, then I go to bed; most of the time, I don't fall asleep, but the sereneness of my room feels much better than school. I always wonder what the next day will be like, trying to think of something positive, and hoping I feel better soon. Every day. Sometimes I can tolerate the aches, but sometimes, it's just too much – the children and teachers' voices, the principal screaming – all of them echoing inside of my head. I can't help it.

Day after day, I start to feel worse.

"It hurts! My head hurts too much, mami!" I tell her, tired of the pain.

"I'll take you to the hospital, sweetheart."

The Charlestown Medical Centre is the size of a small house, yet it's the perfect fit for the patients and the doctors. There, they prescribe a few pills for me and ask me to return in a week, in case I don't feel any better.

Every day that passes, I feel more and more drained, with no desire to do anything. Mami reads out loud my school subjects because I find it hard to do it myself.

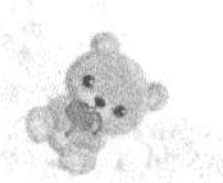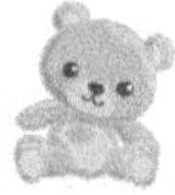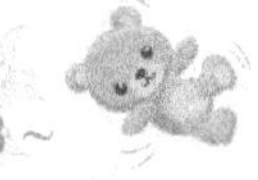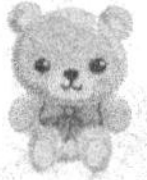

Have I mentioned how much I love her voice? Even my head feels lighter when she talks; besides, I understand everything without a glitch because she finds videos, images, or makes beautiful drawings for me so that every homework seems easy peasy. With my mommy, I learn about so many people and amazing things that I couldn't have with anyone else.

The lesson she taught me about Nelson Mandela was the best. His story really impressed me! From that moment on, I started to become interested in other historic figures, their different roles, and all the strength they spread. My mom teaches me so many different and witty things that it's hard not to like the subjects. It's like she reads tales to me. The truth is, I love home schooling. Here, we can do it in bed, without the irritating noises, or tables, or dumb questions, or people yelling at you. It's so amazing that my body aches barely bother me!

One day, the teachers call mamita again and she takes me straight to the Charlestown Medical Center. But once we get there, they send us to Castlebar's hospital instead, which is way bigger, with lots of doctors and many levels. It's nuts that even though the building is huge, the Barcelona one looks like a skyscraper next to it.

I hate hospitals, especially here. In Spain, at least everyone knows us – the doctors, the other parents, the children (who are my friends), the nurses. We always ended up meeting someone we know. I don't like the idea of being admitted here; not even for a single day.

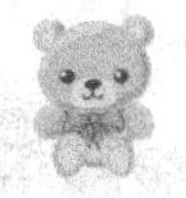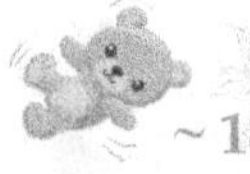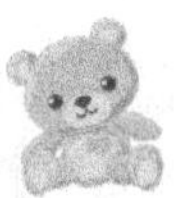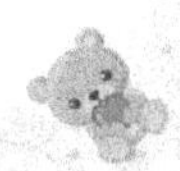

The doctors take me to a small private room where they examine my blood pressure and my temperature over and over again. They also teach me how to rate my headache's intensity using numbers, on a scale from one to ten; it's a bit confusing, but I still get it. You see: one seems almost painless, which is definitely not the case, and ten is too much, might be deadly. Actually, it's very hard to set an exact number because my head hurts quite a lot, but still, I hold on as much as I can. I finally make up a rating, telling the doctors my pain scale is between seven and eight points. That should be ok.

The worst thing about this hospital is the food! For breakfast, they bring me oatmeal, white bread with butter, and hot cocoa. But what's worse is that the beverage is a very, very black tea… that is actually so bitter that it's impossible to drink. Mommy tells me that people in this country like it, and that wherever you go, everyone offers you the same. She says they even mix it with milk and sugar, just like the coffee my teachers in Spain used to drink. Can you imagine something like that? Disgusting! At noon, it's either boiled potatoes or carrots, chicken or fish, a soup, and sometimes an ice cream. For dinner, I have two pieces of toast with butter, plain yoghurt and that horrible tea once more. Everything here has an awful taste! I miss mamita's delicious meals!

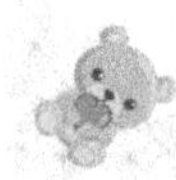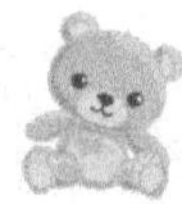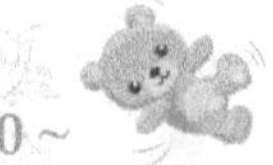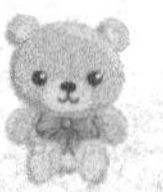

The doctors check up on me daily. They always ask about the pain scale while they write it down on a big notebook and share with the nurses, who, in turn, give me medicines and morphine injections when I need them.

Klim stayed with me, one time, because mamita had to go back to Charlestown to run some errands, take a shower and get some rest. He takes good care of me like a superhero, and also tells me hilarious stories; we have a great time together. The next day, our friend Olga comes with mamita to take him home, so she doesn't have to make a double trip.

THIS PAIN HAUNTS ME

The doctors let us go back home. Even though I've taken all the pills they've given me and my headache went down by at least 3 points on the pain scale, it's still annoying and makes me feel a bit dizzy.

As soon as we go outside, my mommy tells me, "Wow! Feels great to get some fresh air! Do you feel it, dóchenka?"

Even though I don't, I suddenly feel some water drops fall on my face, which was followed by a fresh breeze.

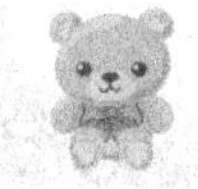 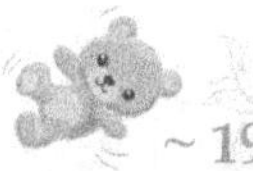 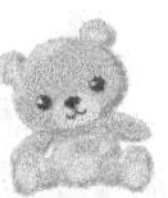 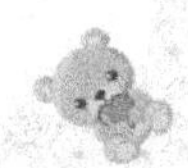

"Yes, mommy. This is much better than the hospital environment!"

That's true. The wind pushes me as I walk, and the drizzle doesn't soak me, at all. It's nice being free from the smell of medicines, alcohol or chlorine. Plus, people walk around wearing colorful clothes, and I think to myself "everything will be alright". My mommy and I take one last look at the hospital before getting in the car.

Seeing her happy is the best feeling in the world.

Klim is already waiting for us when we arrive home. I was anxious to eat whatever I wanted, and sleep in my own big, soft bed with a warm blanket; now, no one will wake me up every hour to take my temperature, or give me injections or pills. Being home is a luxury!

The next day, I'm able to go back to school, but my ache is never at zero. It feels like it's haunting me and I don't know how to get rid of it. Some days, it is usually between three and five on the pain scale. On other days, I'm not so lucky and it starts going higher and higher.

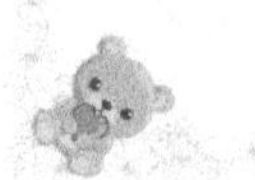
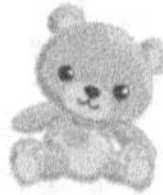
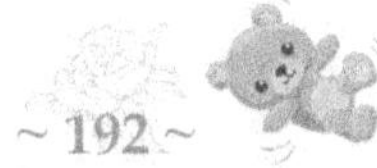
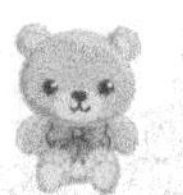

My mommy makes a board to record each medicine she gives me. It kind of reminds me of the one where we wrote down my routine during my chemo; she even drew a lot of mini-squares to mark every single pill I'll be taking during the day. The doctors in Ireland call them "painkillers". In Spanish, it would be something like "pastillas matadolores", but my oncologists from Barcelona don't call them that, but simply "calmantes". Every time I take one, we mark the day and time on the chart. Then we have to wait at least an hour for the next one. Sometimes, the headaches appear ahead of time, and I have no choice but to bite my tongue because the doctors are very strict about respecting the waiting period. I have different pills of all colors, and mami bought morphine too, which used to be a pretty effective painkiller for me, but not anymore. Anyway, the best thing is that we not only have it in the IV form, but also in pills, which is easier for us.

MY DADDY IS HERE!

One day, my mommy leaves the house very early. "Where are you going?" I ask her right away.

"Po delám."

My mommy answers like that sometimes; it means she has to solve some adults' matters.

"I'll be back soon."

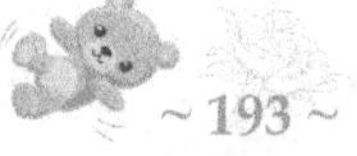
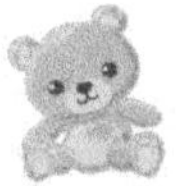
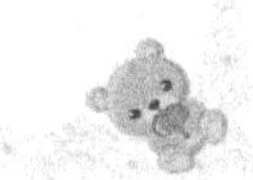

And she did return, in a flash, saying she has a big surprise for me.

"What's the surprise, mommy?"

"You'll see."

My daddy appears out of nowhere. What?! So my mommy went to look for him?! Was that the "matter"?! It's not fair that she hadn't told me anything.

After thinking about it for a while, I feel sad instead of being happy. Why did they keep it a secret? However, my daddy is the funniest man on the planet. He usually makes the best jokes that make me burst out laughing, and listening to them here, again... I'm just glad to have him around. It's weird that he's in Charlestown since he's never been here before, and it's even weirder seeing him home. I gave up my room for him – the one that used to belong to Pavel. It's always better for me to sleep with my mommy anyways. We don't have problems with finding space in this house, you know? Here, there are lots of mattresses for when the family visits, so that everyone has a place to rest.

My headache never goes lower than three points, and mami keeps marking the number of the pain scale on the board, along with the medicines I'd already taken.

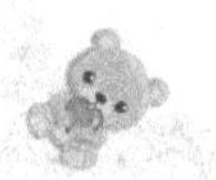
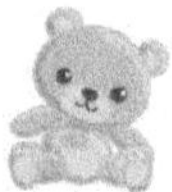
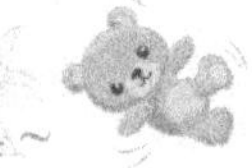
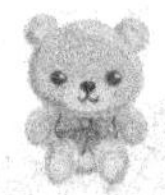

Each hour for my pills gets highlighted one by one, but by this point, there are times when I can't wait for the next dose. The pain has been getting worse faster. Mommy always cheers for me, asking me to hold on a little bit longer, but the truth is that I can't. It's too much for me to handle.

"Mamita!!! Mamita it hurts!! I can't take it!!"

"There's not much time left, baby, let's hold on a little longer."

But she ends up giving me the painkillers early.

My parents are very worried. Mamita offers to go for walks with me. She tells me that some fresh air will help me feel better, so we go out every chance we get, even though I don't feel like doing anything at all most of the time.

On one of these mornings, mami escapes to Spain for a couple of days to sort out some things, while my daddy stays with us to take care of Klim and I. He prepares our food and since his favorite is soup, there's plenty of soup being made. I honestly don't like it. Mommy's dishes are much better. I also know daddy cooks very well because whenever I visit him, we make his signature rectangular pizzas that are finger-licking good. I don't understand why it's not possible here, but I won't think much about that either. We have a great time together either way. My daddy drives us to school and then picks us up, until mamita gets back.

One day, I suddenly feel such a terrible ache that I can't stop screaming. No pill helps me, and it gets stronger by the minute.

"It hurts, Mommy!!! It hurts so much!!! I can't take it anymore, mamita!!! I WANT TO DIE! I want to die already!!! I want to be dead so I don't suffer anymore!!!"

I wish for it with all the strength I have left. That might be the only option to get rid of this pain, so I start hitting my head against the wall to make it disappear. I don't even know how to describe the headache, or which number to give it from one to ten.

My parents try to calm me down so that I stop hurting myself so bad.

"Easy, sweetheart. Be patient, please... everything will be alright, you will be able to take the next dose soon and the pain will go away. You'll see, honey, trust us... You'll see..." they repeat over and over again, hugging me and kissing me all over my face, but I keep crying so much that I feel like I could drown in my own tears.

In the end, once I get tired, I feel the pain start to reduce. One thing or another made it stop, or maybe it was because I fell asleep... I really don't know anything, but this is the worst day of my life.

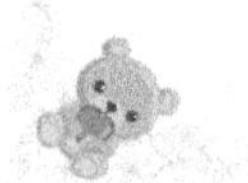
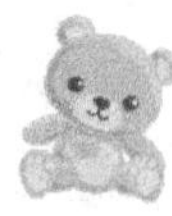
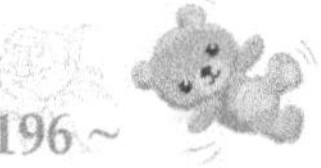
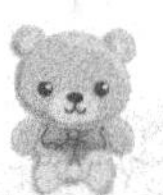

When I wake up in the morning, I stay at home until midday, and once I feel slightly better, I go to school for a couple of hours. With so many pills, I feel dazed though.

My daddy met the new members of the school: Mrs. principal Hart and Mr. assistant principal Bones. He nicknamed the man "Sr. Huesos" because that's what it translates to in Spanish. Now I giggle every time I see them, even though they are bitter and keep screaming every second. It seems to me that those people don't like children... or is it the children who don't like them? Whatever, who knows? The thing is that none of us can stand them. Mr. Bones is also our computing teacher and he gets mad at me if I don't understand something he says, or if I take too long to turn on the computer... sometimes it just doesn't turn on for some reason, and he yells at me in front of the whole class, even though it's not my fault; then my headache gets stronger. I get into trouble whenever I don't hand him my homework on time. Maybe he's also getting annoyed because I often miss out on many of his lessons. The thing is, he screams so much that it feels like the windows would explode, and so does my head.

"Kate, why don't you turn on the computer?! If you don't, I won't let you use it anymore!"

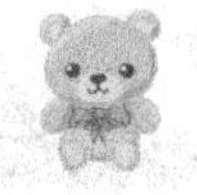 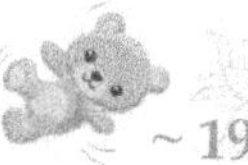 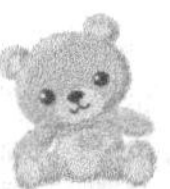 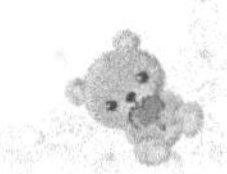

And since the computer won't do what I command, the grumpy man punishes me by cutting off my access. So I sit in class doing nothing, which makes me cry and feel even worse. All my classmates stare at me... like I'm some kind of idiot!

I tell my parents what happened as soon as I get home. I tell them that the vice principal mistreats me, so they decide to go talk to him and Mrs. Hart right away. The next day during my computing class, I can't believe it – it seems that Mr. Bones is no longer Mr. Bones, but his non-evil twin brother. I don't recognize him anymore. He says things like "How can I help you Kate?", "Take your time", or "Ask me for help whenever you need it", and so on, and so forth. I don't know what my parents talked about with him, but I'm sure they said something that made him change beyond recognition. Amazing! I can't wait to get home and tell my parents.

"Mr. Huesos sounds like a different person now, or better yet... An angel! Today, he offered me all the help I needed and even turned on my computer himself, ahead of time. What a relief that he's no longer the monster he used to be. How did you do it?"

"Sometimes people don't see things clearly enough, so we have to help them a bit. Do you see how our conversation helped?"

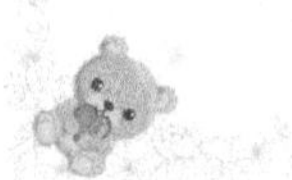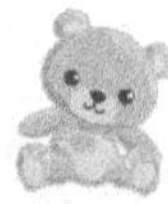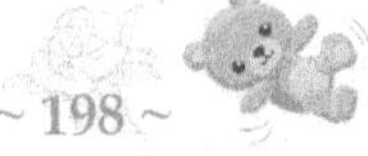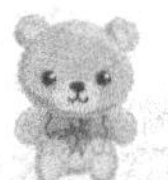

We are really happy. Computing has become my favorite subject now. I get excited about his class and like that he is nice to me. Mr. Bones is the second best teacher in the world; you already know who has the first spot since no one will ever replace McDermott! EVER!

The school also assigned me two support teachers who'll be staying with me all day long. I feel safe. They sit next to me in class, help me carry my backpack when it's heavy, copy my homework from the blackboard because I don't have such a quick hand to do it myself, lend me their smartphones to take a few pictures; during exams, they accompany me to an empty room so that I can concentrate, and I can even dictate the answers while they write them down for me. Although the school is not that big, it has an elevator that only one other girl who is visually impaired, and I, can use; each of us with our aids, whom we secretly call "bodyguards". We are the closest thing to celebrities. I've never been alone since then, nor can anyone mistreat me; nevertheless, I can't help thinking I wish I had friends my same age, and sometimes sadness overcomes me because I don't.

Mamita always tells me, "Don't worry, princess. If you don't have one now, it's because a very special one will show up when you least expect it; when you have a friend, it will last for life, you'll see dóchenka. Besides, I will always be your best friend."

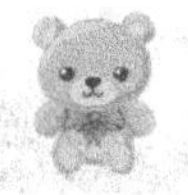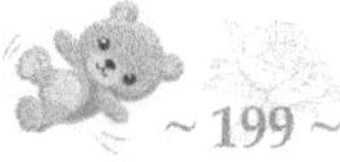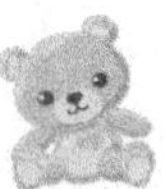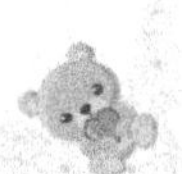

She always speaks to me in Russian, and although I've never been to Russia, I understand her perfectly. I will travel there some day. My brothers and I used to talk in Spanish all the time, but now, after living here for many years, we started speaking in English among ourselves. Well, all of us, except my mommy. If we tell her something in a different language, she corrects us right away. "Tell me the same in Russian, please."

The day of my daddy's departure is coming up and we will have to say goodbye to him soon. I don't think he wants to leave because his face is sad, as if he were about to cry. After he leaves, we are left with our usual daily routine: me going through my headaches, while my mommy and Klim worry about me, helping in whatever they can.

BABULIA'S SURPRISE

As time goes by, it gets harder for me to handle this situation. Mami and I go for a walk in the neighborhood, but we have to take a break every few meters; my legs don't respond. I practically have to drag them to keep going, my body aches don't stop and I almost always have to rest my head on my mommy's shoulder, who never tires of cheering me up.

We take a walk towards downtown, but I feel weaker than usual and tell her, "Let's go home, mamita! I'm tired!"

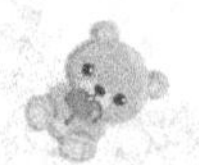
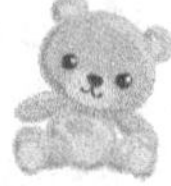
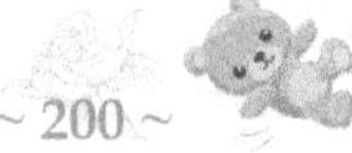
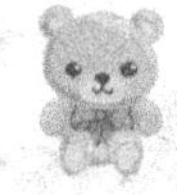

"Just a bit more and we'll turn around."

"Ok."

I don't pay much attention since I have to concentrate on making my legs walk. We finally walk for some more blocks before I tell her again, "Let's go home, mami! I'm tired, let's get back!" hoping she will listen to me.

"Resist a bit more, dóchenka, just a bit. We'll cross the street and then we'll go home."

"Okay."

My head hurts more and more with every step we take, so much so that I can't even see anything around me. I really want to end this walk. My mommy suddenly stops, looking at something. I don't take much notice of it and keep walking, not wanting to raise my head. I already know Charlestown by heart and there is nothing new to see. I could walk around the whole town blindfolded, if I wanted to.

I suddenly see a pair of feet in front of me, but it's strange... those are not my mommy's, since she's standing next to me. Why did this person come so close? I look up slowly to see who it is and..... Oh my God! What do I see?! I can't believe my own eyes!! It's my granny, it's my granny!!! WOW! Babulia?! It is really her?!

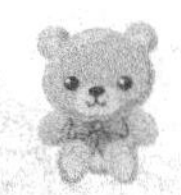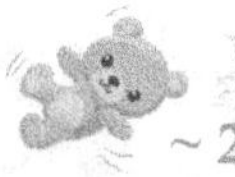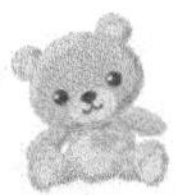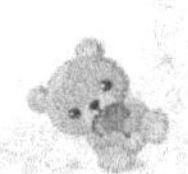

"Babulia! Babulia!" I scream in excitement after realizing what has happened. I have mixed feelings of joy, fright, surprise, I don't know what else, all at the same time. I hug her as hard as I can, sobbing. I feel like the happiest girl in the whole world. What else could I want at this moment, than to have my granny with me?

"Katusha! Katusha!" That's what she calls me. In Russian, it's a sweet version of my name. I love the way it sounds since it makes me feel so loved.

"¡Ya zdes sólnishko, zdes!" which means "I'm here, my sunshine" in Russian. She hugs me tightly as she says that to me.

"Babulia! How did you get here?! Why... b-b-but how... Why didn't you tell me you were coming?" I wonder how all this happened. It seems like a dream.

"I wanted to surprise you, Katusha, I was missing you so much I wanted to see you as soon as possible!"

That is a big surprise for me. A miracle! Being with my granny is like a fairy tale, because she's special, like real life magic. I love her with all my heart!

We walk back home, holding each other. I don't want to be away from my babulia, not even for a second. Mami asks me about the ache, but I tell her that I'm fine. I give a big zero on the scale this time, which is weird, but I don't care. I'm with my granny; that's all that matters to me now. Maybe happiness is the real cure. She is here, and she'll be staying with me for a whole week!

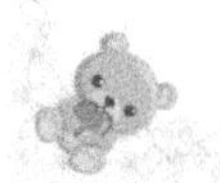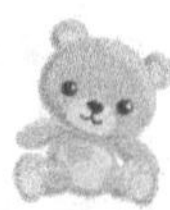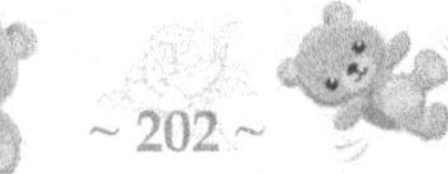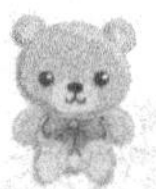

One day, we go shopping in County Mayo. There is a giant Penneys in Ballina town that babulia loves. It has two huge levels with beautiful stuff – more than the one in Spain. I guess it's because this shop is Irish, or so my mommy said. Anyway, it's great to go there with them. We always find what we're looking for, and since it's not expensive, we can buy thousands of things at once: clothes, shoes, utensils, whatever; sometimes we even walk around for hours without getting tired. It's very exciting! Besides, the good Penneys offers can't be missed out, so we buy everything for everyone.

My granny is a school teacher since she likes children. She knows a lot of fun games, which is the reason I like to miss school when my granny stays with us. We also cook some tasty Russian dishes – pelmeni or pirozhki being her specialty, and I love helping her.

Next to our house, on the way to school, is an old train stop. Just on the right side of the road. A hidden path leads to a small abandoned train station where the rails are broken, rusty, and deformed, and all along the track there's green, grass-covered fields, next to a forest. It's beautiful. That's where mamita and I usually take a walk when she picks me up from school. We bump into a bunch of scared little bunnies that run away when they see us. I would like to catch at least one, but they are too fast; even though we try not to scare them, they just run all over the place.

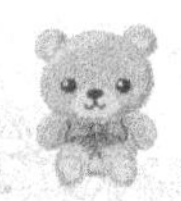
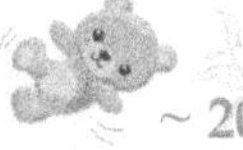
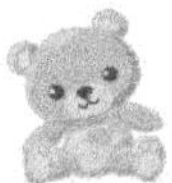
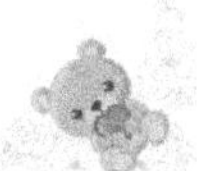

Every now and then, we come across a horse tied up by the tracks. It's kind of scary because he's tied using a very long rope and we don't know how to evade him. We always try to mislead it so we can run away as fast as we can, with our hearts racing; then we laugh at having succeeded. It's hilarious!

Mami loves this route. We call it "the secret doorway" because there are no car noises or people; just the sound of birds singing. Sometimes we even walk barefoot through the grass, which is a bit cold, and almost always wet, but our feet never gets dirty. Babulia also likes being inside that world of nature; she says it reminds her of her childhood. For me, seeing everything green with the magical aura makes me think we are in an enchanted forest.

My pain suddenly comes back, out of the blue, and its much stronger this time. It's awful. I hate it! Some days I stay at home, and on some others, I can go to school but not for so long; the noises and shouting in the classroom gets disturbing. I don't understand why they can't talk in a softer tone. They get so loud I have to yell at them sometimes to be quiet.

Babulia will be flying back to Spain, but I don't want her to leave. If it was up to me, she would live with us forever. We take her to the bus stop, and for the rest of the way, I can't stop thinking of ways to make her stay.

"You must go on," my granny says to all of us. Then she stares at me and continues, "Everything will be fine, Katerina. You just have to keep being the brave and strong, little girl, like you have always been."

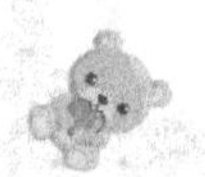 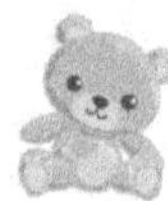 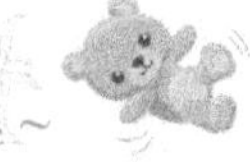 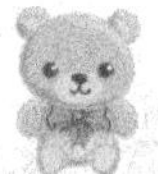

I can feel the tears coming out of my eyes on hearing that. Babulia is the sweetest person, along with my mommy. What would I do without them?

"And you, Klim, take care of your family, you are the man of the house now."

She continues talking to my brother and mom, "Dóchenka… I know you will make it."

She wishes us luck, and then gets on the bus, sitting near a window. It's sad watching her leave. We wave our hands until the bus disappears completely from our sight.

NEW DISCOVERINGS

It's December 2014. I've been suffering for more than a month – a month that seems like an eternity. Day after day, I feel worse, with my headaches rating at the top of the pain scale. In fact, it doesn't even fit since it has already reached one hundred points. It hurts a ton!

One day, my mommy says, "Honey! I've found great solutions to make you get better faster, much faster from now on. Soon we'll remove all the medicines, but we have to do it carefully. I'm sure we'll succeed, you'll see."

"What are you talking about, mamita?"

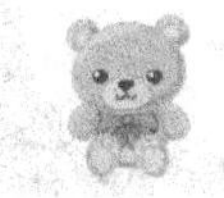
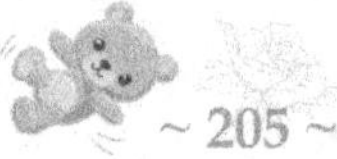
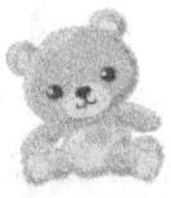
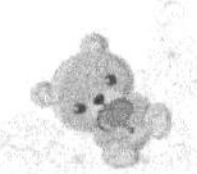

"It's difficult to explain in a nutshell... there are natural treatments without side effects." Her eyes are shining, like she has a brilliant idea.

I want to get out of this situation now. I've been suffering not only from the headaches, but many other things have added up till now: my belly is swollen and sore, I have eczemas on my arms – sometimes under my eyes. My fingers are swollen too, and it hurts if I bend them so I can't even write. My hands and feet are also white as a sheet. They are always icy-cold and I don't feel them.

"Your daddy sent me a video of a medical conference where they talk about completely different treatments, and it's barely known these days. The first thing we need to do is focus on our diet."

I have no idea what this diet change means!

"We are going to eat differently from now on," she goes on.

My brother and I look at her with wide eyes, trying to understand what it's going to be like to eat differently since we already eat healthy. That doesn't sound good at all; is she going to stop cooking yummy meals??? I honestly don't like the idea.

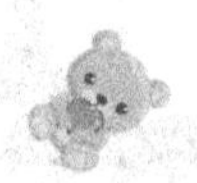 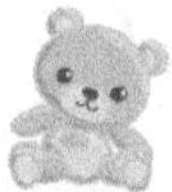 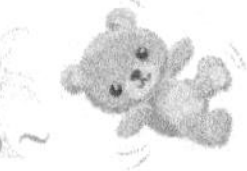 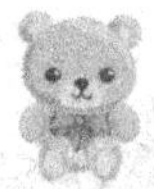

Then she keeps telling us, "We are going to use some specific plants that attack the tumor, and don't harm your health as they are natural; that, along with other things that help you recover faster."

We pay attention to what she's saying, hoping to see where the magic trick is.

"From now on, every single thing we eat is going to be organic, and I'll prepare only chicken and fish two or three times a week."

That is how we started our new diet. Organic food is actually good, but it's ten times more expensive and three times smaller, so my mommy doesn't cook chicken or fish every day, and when she does, she serves us smaller portions. Red meat has been completely erased from our menu, but I don't care because I've never been a fan. Whenever I go to my daddy's house, he gives me a huge steak for dinner that I can never finish… or rather, I can't even start, since it's bigger than my face. Most of the time, I feed it to the cats he has at home when he's not watching. Luckily, I don't have to eat it now.

Mami keeps telling us about it, "I have to buy wild fishes because they don't have hormones nor chemicals."

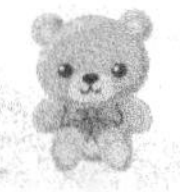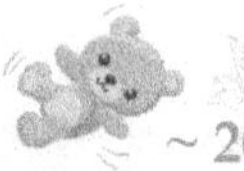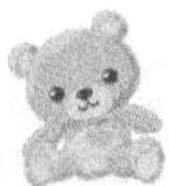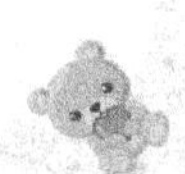

WOW! I didn't know that animals had so many things in their bodies... I didn't notice. They look delicious! We didn't even have time to get used to our new, low meat diet when my mommy gives us some more news.

"No! No! No! I've made a mistake, kids. Let's make another change. Now we'll follow the macrobiotic diet, which is healthier than the other one."

That sounds very scientific.

"Mommy, what does a macro... biotic diet mean?" we ask her.

"It's when you don't eat chicken – only fish, plus fruits, vegetables, seeds, beans and legumes."

She seems happy about not having to buy that expensive chicken that she didn't like cleaning.

As we slowly get used to the macrobiotic diet, mami surprises us one more time. "No! No! I'm wrong again, kids. It's not the macrobiotic diet that we need; the vegetarian one is much better. And we also have to say goodbye to gluten."

Klim and I know what that is, but what does the other one mean?

"And what is this ve-ge-tarian diet?"

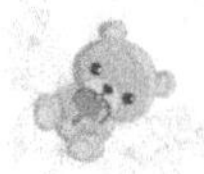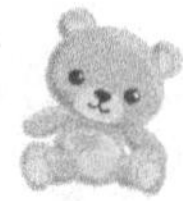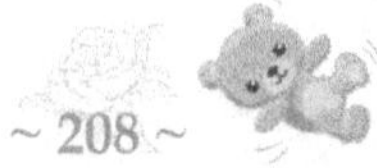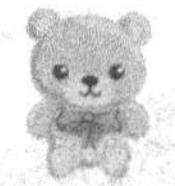

"*Vegetarian means that from now on, we cannot eat meat of any kind; not even processed meat.*"

"*What is processed meat, mom?*" *Klim asks.*

"*They are products made from the meat of animals that were once alive, then killed and converted into a new product. These dead animals are like corpses, not healthy for our bodies.*"

"*Poor things,*" *I tell my mommy right away.* "*I love animals, I don't want them to be killed.*"

"*Neither do I, honey. We won't eat them anymore.*"

"*We are not going to eat animals!*" *I say out loud.*

"*And the sausages, bologna, hams or hamburgers are out too.*"

"*WHAT?! Why mommy?*" *Klim asks.*

"*Because it's also made from processed animals. This meat goes through a crushing machine that turns them into some kind of mash, then they add more unhealthy things.*"

"*And what about the sausages we like so much? The ones that we buy at LIDL, the German smoked and fatty ones that are so yummy... We are not going to buy them either?*"

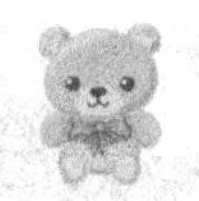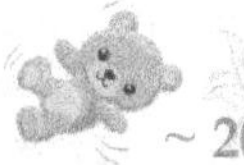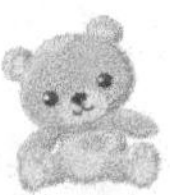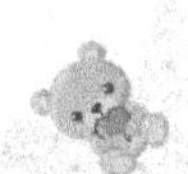

"No, baby. We are not going to buy them anymore. Do you remember how greasy they get when I cook them?" We nod with eyes wide open. "Well, that fat is the main content of the sausages and what makes them so good... but it harms our body."

"But mommy... they're so good... and you like them too!"

"Yes, it's true baby, they are delicious... but we used to buy them because I didn't know how they were made. Now I know. They are made up of so many things that you can't even imagine."

"And the hamburgers? We are not even going to eat hamburgers anymore?" Klim asks her in a tone that goes from being sad to annoyed.

"Never again," my mommy sentences.

"It's not fair, mommy! I want my burgers, everybody eats them! You can't do this to me! I want to eat them!" Klim yells, runs up to his room and slams the door.

Truth be told, I don't care. But hamburgers... those are good. Oh gosh! Klim is right, but if my mommy says not to do something, whatever it is, I have to listen to her. Besides, I want to heal and forget about these aches for once.

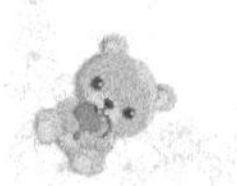 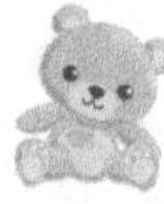 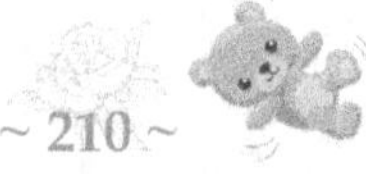 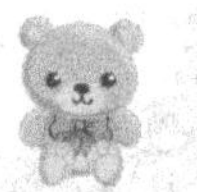

"I don't want to eat dead animals! I don't like that... Why did we eat them before, mamita?" I keep questioning her, while imagining how we could eat something like that. I can't even think of cow or chicken corpses on my plate... Yuck! It's disgusting!

"Honey, we used to eat it because everybody does; no one questions it or looks for the information about it, but I already have. I'm going to show you more details step by step. You'll see, honey. They have discovered many things in different labs, universities and scientific centers," I'm shocked, although I don't understand much.

The next day mommy tells us, "I was serious yesterday when I told you that we will stop eating meat, sausages and hamburgers. In fact, we will not only stop eating those, but all processed food in general."

"There's other processed food? What is that?" my brother and I ask, interested.

"It's all the food that goes through a process of preparation and cooking...in other words, it's more or less cooked already. Then they add additive stuff like chemicals, preservatives and colorants, plus tons of sugar and very low quality salt to make it last longer in the supermarkets. With all these procedures, many good things are lost from the products, such as vitamins, minerals and enzymes. I'll tell you which ones they are. Are you ready?"

"Yes please! Tell us, mommy. Tell us already." Klim looks scared; he doesn't seem to be expecting good news.

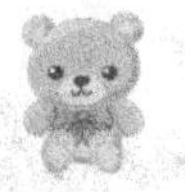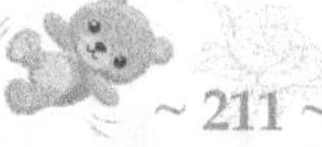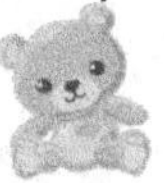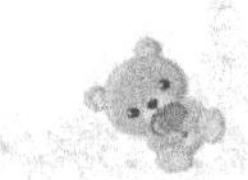

"These are ketchups, sodas, frozen foods, pizzas, ice cream, all products made of flour such as breads, buns, croissants... although I love them... biscuits, chocolates, sweets, everything that's bottled and packaged."

Just hearing the first two on the list, my brother Klim panics right away.

"NOOO! Mom, no! I don't want you to take away the ketchup and soda! I can't live without them... So, what are we going to drink now anyways?"

"We can make iced tea infusions, or just water, which is much healthier."

"Yuck! Water and tea?!" Klim and I answer at the same time.

"They are not yummy at all! And water is tasteless..." Klim keeps complaining angrily.

"We'll get used to it. Besides, I'm going to introduce natural drinks made of fresh fruit, which are delicious and much better for our bodies. We are going to prepare them ourselves... and not just from oranges, we can make juice out of a wide variety of fruits and vegetables, using a special machine that I'll buy soon."

Ouch! I don't like this at all. Orange juice is disgusting, and its pulp is annoying.

"Nobody eats like that, mom. I want my ketchup and soda!"

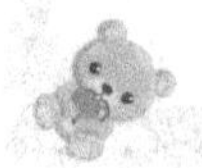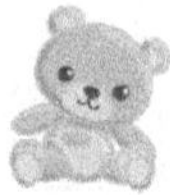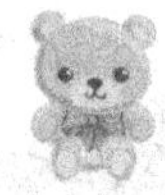

"Ok, Klim, let's make a deal then... so you don't feel so bad about this. We'll buy one bottle of ketchup per week, instead of one every two days, and it won't be thirty bottles of soda a month anymore, but only two. If you run out too quickly, you'll have to wait until the next purchase. We're good with it?"

My brother loves ketchup. He adds tons of it to every meal, and no food has taste for him if he doesn't. I don't find it pleasant to add ketchup to everything; only if it's something I don't like. Mommy and Klim came to a pact to buy very little, although he's not into it. Even so, my brother keeps finishing his stuff as quickly as before, maybe hoping that a miracle will happen and they'll reappear out of nowhere.

He probably thinks that one day, mamita will anticipate the purchase, but every time Klim mentions that he doesn't have his ketchup or his soda, mamita's answer remains the same, "You already know how it works, Klim, it's not your shopping day yet."

"Hooooo nooooo!" Klim answers in despair and keeps eating without his favorite things.

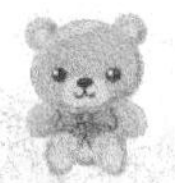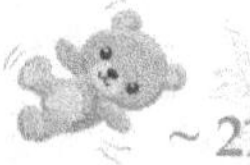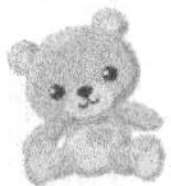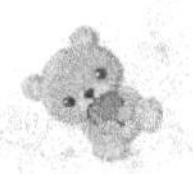

Mommy learns how to make delicious ketchup so that Klim doesn't suffer so much. It's more like a tomato paste which is much better and nutritive... nothing like the one we used to buy. She asks me if I have a new notebook to write down her healthy recipes, so I give her a school diary that I've never used. The "yummy ketchup" was the first one; we named it that because it's fabulous. Klim hardly remembers the supermarket's bottle anymore, nor does he find it tasty. Mamita is very happy because my brother now prefers her homemade ketchup.

Every day my mommy teaches us what these changes in our diet mean. During all the time we have kept away from meat, hamburgers, IKEA meatballs, or LIDL sausages, mommy explains to us why it's better to substitute them with vegetables, showing us videos about it, making us realize that we used to put harmful things into our bodies.

I trust her. Sometimes I get distracted by all the information she hands us, or rather, I don't understand everything as well as Klim. It's perhaps because of my lack of energy. During some moments, mami asks us to pay attention carefully. The worst thing is that she asks us questions about those videos, and if we don't know the answer, she repeats them again and again until we have it memorized. Now we know that we must be more attentive so that we don't have to watch the same videos too many times.

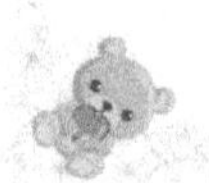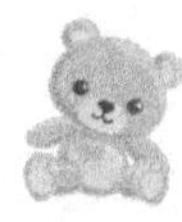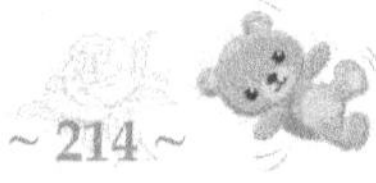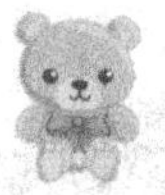

She also reads us some curious facts over and over again, shows us pictures so that we can ask her anything we can think about, and have no doubts left. It's hard not to learn everything mamita teaches us.

Our favorite dishes are slowly starting to disappear from the table and the diet is becoming more and more bland. We eat lots of beans and vegetables, and there's not much variety... it's boring. The cabinets no longer stock the delicious things they used to, and it doesn't matter how much we search for them in the whole house, we don't find anything what we want – only tons of fruits and vegetables, either in the fridge or in every corner of the house. We eat salads every day, like we always do, but for the second meal, we now have things like quinoa, buckwheat, red or black rice, legumes or potatoes with vegetables along with more... vegetables. That's it! Vegetables, vegetables, and more vegetables... everywhere! Until the broccoli sprouts out of my ears! Vegetables in our salads, vegetables as a main dish, fruits for dessert. We eat huge meals, but always remain hungry. I don't enjoy that food; besides, I despair at the thought that even with all the changes we've made, I still feel awful.

We started a new treatment at the same time as this diet change. It's called Homeopathy. Mami has reduced the number of traditional pills, and started to introduce some small, sweet balls that are made from medicinal plants.

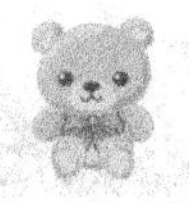
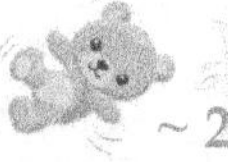
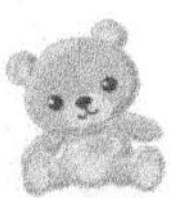
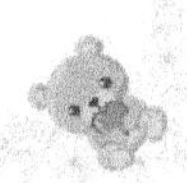

She wants us to make these changes slowly so that we can get rid of morphine and other strong medications. These plants have been prescribed to me by Dr. Prasanta Banerji, a very famous doctor from India; he gave mommy a procedure specially designed for me. She looks very happy when she talks to me about it, and of course, I am too.

One day, mamita gives us some other news about our diet.

"I have some news, kids. Our actual diet is not the one we should follow. I made a mistake. We should be vegan."

"Vegan??!! What is that? Isn't that the same as being a vegetarian?" Ouch! Right when we'd already learned that word… and they kind of sound the same!

"Being a vegan is about not only avoiding animals, but anything produced by them. That means no eggs or dairy products. Also, our food has to be divided into a mix which is at least half cooked and half raw."

I don't really know about this vegan thing, but it seems like we have to take out way more stuff… what a pity!

"Another change, Mamita? Why?" Klim asks.

"Animal products aren't easy to digest, and that affects our health."

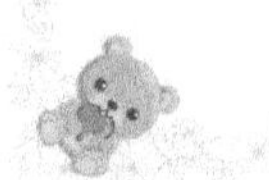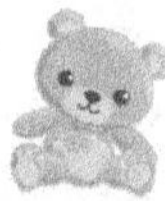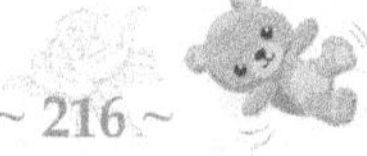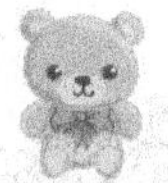

"What are dairy products?" we ask at the same time.

"Dairy products are made from milk, such as butter, mayonnaise, ice cream, yoghurts and cheese."

"Cheese?! What do you mean, no cheese, Mami?! They're delicious!!! Why Mommy?" Klim insists, getting sad again. "And what are we going to put on the bocatas we take to school? If we don't eat ham, no bread, and not even cheese now."

"Yes mamita... What will the bocatas be like now? Without cheese, ham, nor the bread that we like." Bocatas are Spanish ham and cheese sandwiches... How do we make a bocata without ham and cheese? I can't believe she suddenly took everything away from us.

"What are we going to put inside what? What are we going to eat now?" Klim complains.

"Don't worry guys, we'll find an alternative to replace it all. There will surely be something tasty to use; we just have to discover it. Oh! Another thing is that we can't buy chocolates anymore."

"What?! Chocolates too?" Well, that was a low blow. This diet is the worst! "Mamita, what are you talking about? Why? Not the chocolate, please! How can you take it away from me?"

My mommy hit a sensitive nerve of mine – having to say goodbye to the only yummy thing I had left...

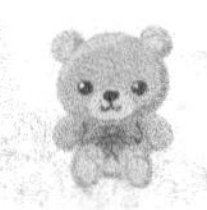 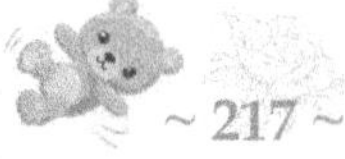 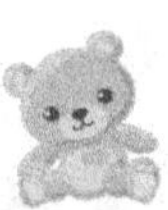 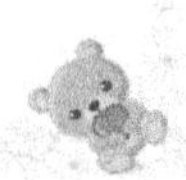

"I don't want to, mommy!" I tell her, trying to hold back my tears, then the headache becomes stronger. I don't care about ketchup, soda, or hamburgers, but chocolate?!!! NOOOO!!

She throws more details, "The chocolates, princess, have milk. Almost all the chocolates in the market have milk, and milk is the main culprit of your skin allergies, that's why we have to remove it. Your eczemas will disappear once we remove milk from our diet. Besides, chocolates also have lots and lots of sugar, and this refined sugar is the cancer cells' favorite food. They love it and eat it all, growing and multiplying with an extraordinary speed. Since they are such gluttons, they need twenty times more sugar than any healthy cell in our body... we can't keep feeding them, can we, Katerina?"

"That's right, mamita," I end up answering, full of sadness. "I don't want to feed them, and I don't want them to grow, or multiply, or hurt me anymore... but I don't want chocolate to disappear from our lives either."

"I understand, honey, but we have to cut their food source. Look at it like this: we'll educate the cancer cells and give them healthy food so that they can become healthy cells again, that's how they used to be anyways. Then they'll have two options; to die if they don't want to learn anything about food, or to survive and become your friends. They decide for themselves, but we have to be good teachers so that they learn well. What do you think?"

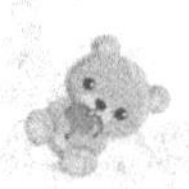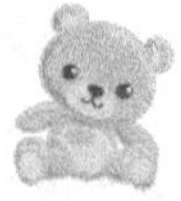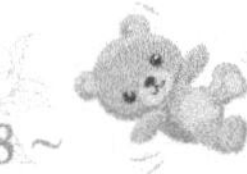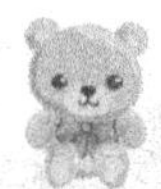

"Interesting! I like being a teacher, so I'm going to show them how to become my friends. Just like at school."

"We can do a lot of things to help them behave, like giving them lots of oxygen to make them healthy – fresh food, for example."

I don't like my mommy's idea, at first, but then it starts to sound exciting. Maybe, when the cancer is well-behaved, I will be able to eat my chocolate again? Who knows?

Mami makes lots of cooking discoveries every day, and tries to prepare enjoyable things for us. For the first few weeks, the food was boring and repetitive, almost always the same. But suddenly, we started to eat differently, with many more grains, and many, many more vegetables, some fruits, seeds, and nuts. Now my mommy even makes the bread; it's not white, like the one we used to buy at the supermarket, or big enough to cut. It's like a round bun with curved edges… like a flat cupcake. In fact, we use the muffin molds for the bread since my mommy can't buy some new ones. This new bread that she makes is great – it's soft, with sunflower seeds, sesame, or pumpkin... or all at once. The only thing I don't like much is that it's too dark. As time goes by, we start getting used to it, until there comes a time when we don't remember the other one.

Despite that, the same question pops up again, "And what are we going to put inside this bread mommy?" we keep insisting.

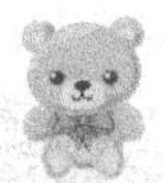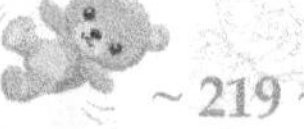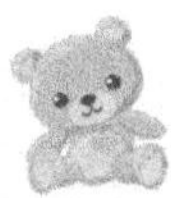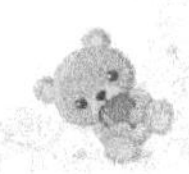

"Don't worry children, we will find the solution, and it will be much better than before. I promise."

Since we can't put anything inside our sandwiches yet, we eat at home together. I can't stay at school all day. Sometimes I don't even go, and since Klim has his bike, he's home in like five minutes to have lunch with mommy and me.

There are some organic shops in Sligo where we find delicious vegan cheeses – they're supposed to be super healthy because they're made out of plants and seeds. Our bocatas are finally back! When we don't have cheese, mamita makes the sandwiches with an avocado cream that she makes by herself, a slice of tomato, some onion, and at times, some lettuce. These vegan dishes are actually fabulous, and "the vibrant tomato ham", as mummy calls it, gives the bocatas a different flavor. We've never eaten them like this before.

My brother's classmates ask him, "Where's your ham, Klim?" His snack looks like something from another planet to them. At home, he tells us his story and we all laugh together.

My brother kept asking mamita for milk, so they made another deal: she told him that she would buy him an organic one, in small quantities, of course. Klim was happy with that, for a while, until one day he stopped taking it and the tetra-Brik stopped coming out of the fridge.

My mommy, surprised, asks him, "Klim, what happened with the milk?"

"I decided not to drink it. I've seen too many documentaries and articles. I don't want it anymore, mom."

"That's my boy! Congratulations! I'm so glad you were able to come to this conclusion on your own."

Nevertheless, the changes we've made to our lifestyle and diet still don't make me feel any better. Mamita always gives me some stuff to ease my aches, but they remain from eight to ten on the pain scale. Or rather... from eighty to one hundred. I hate this pain! It seems to be endless, and I have no choice but to keep holding on.

The doctors haven't left me alone since we left Castlebar's hospital. Some people called "Hospice group" usually stop my house. I don't know what their name means; only that they take care of me, give me my daily dose of morphine and other medicines, and if I'm missing something, they write a new prescription right away. We can call them any time we wanted. I have more bodyguards now! Not only at school, but at home too! Even so, I feel so weak that I can hardly pay attention to them, or the teachers. I want to feel better once and for all.

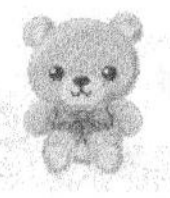
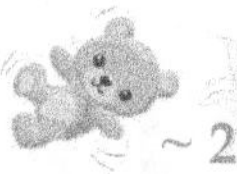
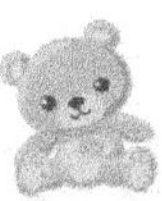
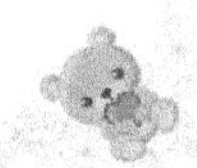

I'm excited because Christmas season is coming soon, and I know that I'll see my cousins, my uncle Ilusha, my granny, and my aunt Liubasha in Spain... Mamita already bought the plane tickets months ago! The doctors-bodyguards don't want us to leave because they worry too much about me, but my mommy manages to convince them. We're going to have medical control in Barcelona anyways, and besides, we can't miss the best holiday of the year. In the end, they let us go, wishing us a good time outright.

"Are you sure you have enough energy for this trip, honey?" she asks me, once the doctors were ok with the plans.

"Yes, yes, yes! Mommy... I'm one hundred percent sure. Let's go! I want to go to Spain!"

I think she's not aware of how anxious I am for the trip. Even though, I don't feel good at all these days, with the headache driving me nuts and no improvement at all... that trip is the only thing that gives me hope.

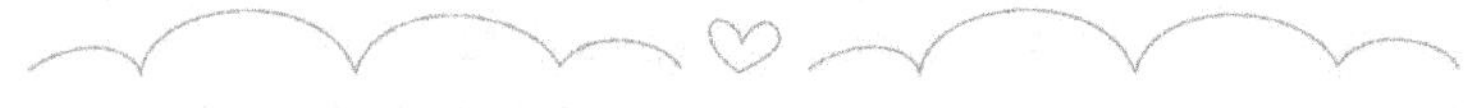

CHRISTMAS IN SPAIN

I feel worse than ever on the day of our flight to Spain. Luckily, the bus stop is only a ten-minute walk away, and my brother helps me carry my bags.

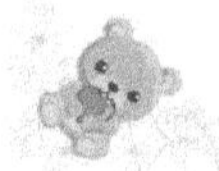
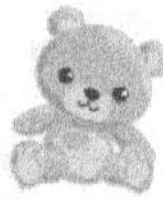
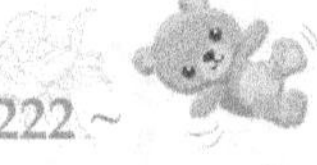
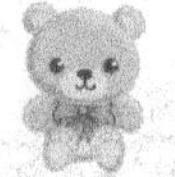

Otherwise I don't think I can make it. I'm giving my best so that we don't stay in Ireland. Klim and I don't play as much as we used to because lately, I've been too sleepy… that makes me really sad. When we get to the bus stop, we have to wait for a while since it's still very early. There are no people on the streets, and the sun hardly rises behind the teeny tiny houses; but it seems to me that the bus is late on purpose. Thank God, it finally arrived. I feel calmer because I will have some rest. Once I'm inside, I'll be able to take a three-hour nap until we get to the airport.

Despite how tired I am, I can't sleep a wink during the whole bus trip. At least, not like I'd expected. We arrive at Dublin's airport, take our direct flight to Barcelona, and in only a couple of hours, we land. I think I was asleep most of the way, but even so, I feel very tired.

My daddy is waiting for us, to take us to my granny's house from the airport, where we are going to spend our Christmas holidays; he brought the magic plants that mommy had asked him for. They say those pills are called "supplements"…weird. Anyways, they give me the pills before we leave for Tarragona and I seem to fall asleep… again. I'm supposed to take them to feel better, but I'm tired of waiting for that improvement to happen. Daddy drives back home after leaving us at my granny's, and I'm happy again. I've missed babulia so much! It feels like I haven't seen her in a long time!

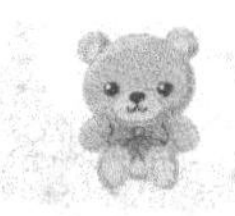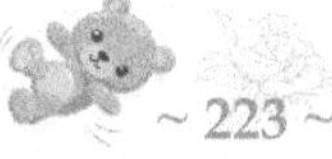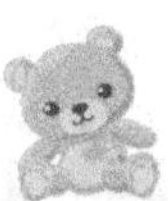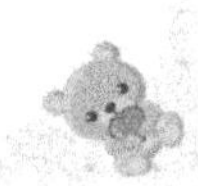

Since we've been on that vegan diet, my swelling has gone down a bit. I still look like a balloon, but maybe eating gluten-free, with half the fruits and vegetables raw, is working after all. Mami also prepares some special baths for me at babulia's house. She uses water from the Mediterranean that she, along with all the men of the house, bring directly from the sea. Actually, we started doing that in Ireland, but in a different way: first mamita bought many, huge buckets full of salt, and then we placed them in the hall next to the bathroom. They were lined up one on top of the other, in rows, up to the ceiling. Here in Spain, they heat up the water first and I stay in the tub for twenty or thirty minutes, with my mommy always by my side, talking sweetly to me. Sometimes she even gets in, hugging me. In other cases, it's babulia who stays there – and every now and then, they both stay with me. These baths are so relaxing that I even fall asleep.

My daddy installs a kind of temporary stove in granny's bathroom so that the sea water can be heated up directly there, in a heavy pot that can't even be lifted. I've never seen a pot this size before! Luckily, this is quite a big bath, so all the stuff they place inside fits quite easily. I'm sure we couldn't do the same in our Ireland house.

Mamita still cooks the vegan dishes, but they are stricter for me than for my brother; he and the rest of my family eat something different.

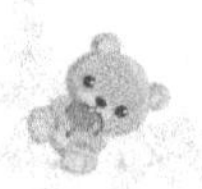 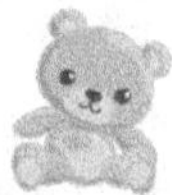 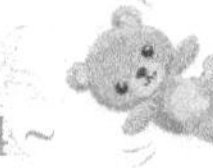 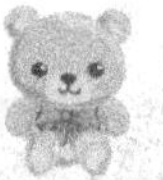

She can't afford that kind of food for all of us, so I'm the only one who gets the organic products. They aren't bad, not at all – they're actually delicious. The thing is that I don't feel like eating anything anymore.

We go for walks almost daily, and both the morphine and the other medicines have been slowly taken away.

Mamita is really excited about it and is constantly encouraging me saying, "When all the pills that harm you are gone, you will only be left with natural things. Be patient, little princess, you will soon get better."

My daddy picks us up and take us on walks along the sea coast in Salou. When I was little, the whole family lived in that city – my granny, my uncle Ilusha, who was still a child, my cousin Adelina, my aunt Liubasha, my mommy and my brothers. I was a year old when we moved from there and it's not like I remember it... I know the stories that the adults tell me. We all lived together in an apartment in front of the sea, until one day when we got divided into three different families and started on different paths.

There are days when I don't feel like going out, but mommy still insists because she thinks that will make me feel better somehow, so I make an effort; however, the only thing I think about when we go for walks is wishing a bench would appear on the way so that I can sit and rest... When will I feel better? My body is a mess; it's very difficult for me... more than they can imagine.

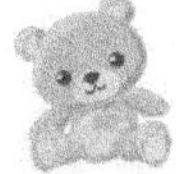

"Baby, we only walked fifty meters. We just got out. A bit more baby, just a little bit," my mommy keeps encouraging me.

"No, mamita… please, let's go back. I don't want to." I'm exhausted. Every step becomes a torture. I want to stop walking, fall on the bench, and never get up.

A TERRIBLE NIGHT

It's Christmas Eve; the night we get together with the whole family. I haven't taken the medicines the doctors gave me in two days. We've replaced them with plants – the ones in the supplements form. These are supposed to be much more powerful and effective, not to mention that they don't have any side effects, and all that stuff my mommy explained to me, but I still feel terrible.

It couldn't be worse.

There's another serious problem now: I can't pee. My belly feels like it's getting tighter and tighter. Whenever I go to the toilet, nothing comes out. The worst thing is that it's been this way since yesterday, accumulating all this liquid inside me. The whole day was horrific and at some point, I fell asleep, until I couldn't take the bellyache much longer.

"Mamita! Mami… my tummy hurts. I want to pee."

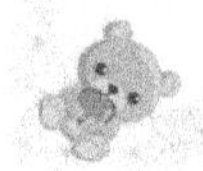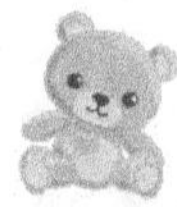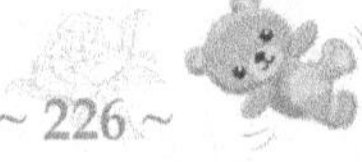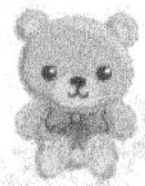

After several tries, she says:

"I'll give you a diuretic infusion that'll help you pee, honey."

We come and go in a flash. I was hoping this infusion would have a quick effect, but then again... nothing. After sitting in the toilet for a while, I get angry with myself and start to cry; it doesn't matter how hard I try, my body isn't working anymore. What should I do to make the pee come out anyways? I don't get it.

My mommy tries to calm me down by telling me that everything will be alright. We spend a few hours between the bathroom and the kitchen, but in the end, she brings a hot bottle and says, "Let's put this on your tummy to help relax the muscle and release the pee. You'll see, baby, it will come out."

We wait, wait, wait... We wait for so long that I end up falling asleep with the bottle on my tummy.

I almost don't fall sleep because I can't stand my bellyache anymore. It's about to explode. When I open my eyes, I see my mommy sitting next to me, waiting for me to wake up, or so it seems. She hasn't slept at all – I can notice it on her face.

A cocktail of aches takes over my body, all of them at once, making my night even worse. I don't know how to describe them exactly. Along with my head and belly aches, I have to face another nightmare: suffocation.

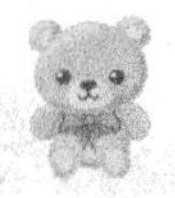 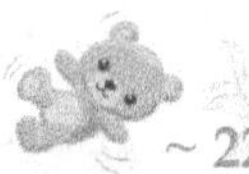 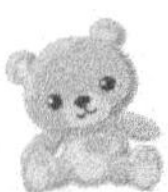 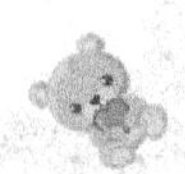

I'm short of breath. I try to tell mamita what's happening to me, but my voice can hardly be heard. It's weird, I don't even have the strength to speak clearly.

"Mamita! Mamita! I can't breathe! Am I dying, mami? I can't! I can't breathe, mamita!"

"Quick! Quick, dóchenka! Let's go get some fresh air by the window! Quick, baby!" My mommy sounds nervous.

I can barely walk, so she lifts me up in her arms to the bathroom's tiny window, where she supports my back. I'm grabbing onto the edges as tight as I can; it's difficult, but I help myself by getting on tippy-toes.

"Breathe, sweetheart, take a deep breath, come on... not like that..."

She shows me what I should do to get my breathing back to normal. "That's it, baby, inhale all you can, exhale... slowly. That's it, honey! You're doing great! Again, breathe in as much air as you can, come on! Again, slowly baby, come on, you can do it!"

My mommy mirrors my actions. I try to breathe slowly, but sometimes I lose control... Suddenly, I feel the air flowing through my lungs and, even though I start feeling a bit dizzy, I keep doing what she tells me.

"Don't stop, baby! That's right... keep going… keep going… good! You're doing great, baby! You're a strong girl, come on! Keep it up… keep it up! Very good..." Her voice makes me regain energy.

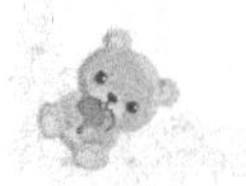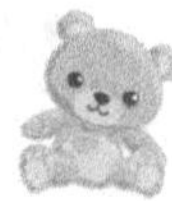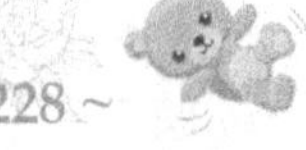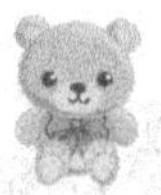

Babulia suddenly appears at the door and starts encouraging me without really knowing what's happening. She runs quickly towards me and stands by the other side, supporting my back, just like mommy does. I feel the air flowing strongly through my body. I'm losing the strength to keep standing, but I remember mamita saying that I'm a strong girl and I hold on to that.

Actually, it got worse. But I must keep going; I will fight until the end.

Though it was just a few minutes of bustling by the bathroom's tiny window, it felt like an entire day to me. I can breathe! I made it!

"Very good, dóchenka! You did very well! You're strong... you're very strong! I know that. I love you, my little princess."

"Very good Katusha!!! Very good!!!"

They hug me carefully once I've recovered. My belly is still swollen... my headache and bellyache seemed to be joined as one. Plus, a warmness runs through my body. What's happening?

"You're going to take the bath right now, we don't have time to waste....we can't wait until the evening. That fever should be lowered," Mami says, after taking my temperature.

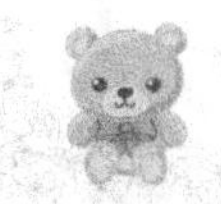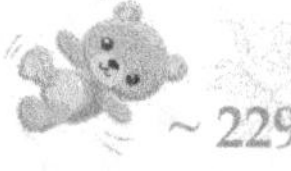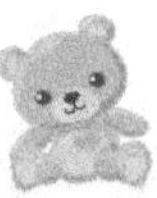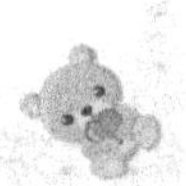

They prepare the bath in a flash. My energy quickly leaves me these days. I'm so weak that I can't feel any part of my body; even my neck can't completely support my head. So I need my mommy and granny's help to raise my feet and get into the water.

Once in the tub, covered up to the neck in salty water, my eyes start closing while babulia holds my head carefully so that I don't slide.

"Go get some rest, dóchka, go to my room. I'll be right here with Katusha, don't worry," I hear my granny's voice fade as I fall asleep in the tub.

My mommy leaves the bathroom and I stay with my granny, who caresses my head, my arms and my legs... saying the sweetest things. I don't really know if I fell asleep or simply closed my eyes for a bit, but it's already time to get out of the tub. Babulia dries me off with a towel and I start feeling a bit too chilly.

"Your fever has gone down, Katusha... quite a lot. Soon you'll feel great again, vnúchenka, you'll see," Babulia says, as she looks at the thermometer.

I start wearing my pajamas when I suddenly feel a strong need to pee... oh my gosh, finally! I think it's going to come out everywhere!

"T-t-toilet..."

That's the only thing I can pronounce... sadly, it seems that I don't even have the energy to talk.

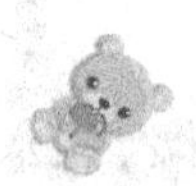 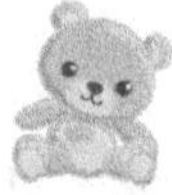 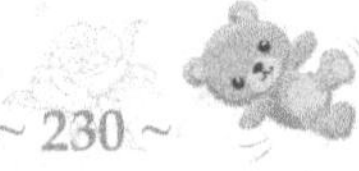 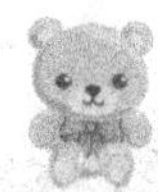

Will I be able to pee this time? Or will it be another false alarm? Babulia helps me sit on the toilet, turns on the bidet, and then sits next to me on the tub's rung.

"This will help you relax. Focus on that sound, Katusha, you'll pee anytime..." I'm dazed and my eyes start to close by themselves. I can't control them at all, but... suddenly...

A jetstream starts gushing into the toilet. It stops, and starts again, stops once more, and starts... until it rushes out with such force that I thought it would shoot me out of the toilet, like a rocket.

"YEEEEEAH!!!! WOW!!!! Katusha!!! Yeah!!! Yeah!!! That's it!!!!!" My granny screams so loud that I think she wakes up everyone in the house, and it makes me want to pee even more.

The pee starts coming out as forceful as a giant waterfall. It feels like my body is slowly deflating. Babulia is jumping with joy, and a few seconds later my mommy opens the door abruptly, with a confused face, looking like she's about to cry.

"What happened?!"

Mommy starts crying with excitement when she understands what's going on... I can't say anything to her because I'm focused on peeing.

"Finally, dóchenka! Keep going… keep going, don't stop! That's it!"

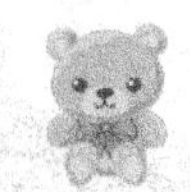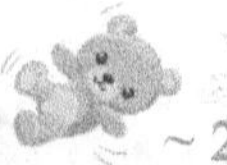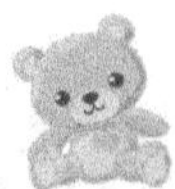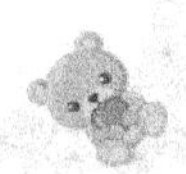

I don't want to stop, and even if I wanted to, I don't think I have control over this waterfall. It comes out with more and more force every second, and while that happens, I notice that my belly is almost completely deflated and the pressure on it is going down. I feel free.

This pee jet is endless. As soon as it stops, the second accumulated batch starts again, and so on for a while. When it's finally over, I remain sitting on the toilet for a few more minutes, just in case. I'm so tired that I could fall asleep right here… I want to go to sleep so badly.

As my mommy and my granny help me get to my feet, a painful cramp in my belly hits me so hard that it makes me scream.

"What happened?! What happened, baby?!" My mommy is holding me tight so I don't fall. This time, I don't want to pee, not at all; there's something bigger behind this pain.

"T-t-toilet… to-toi-let…" A rough diarrhea takes me by surprise.

Even though I'm cold, my body is covered in sweat. Everything repeats over and over again. This is exhausting…

"I can't take it anymore! I can't! I want it to stop now! Why doesn't it stop? I'm in pain… mamita."

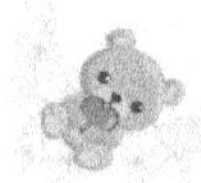
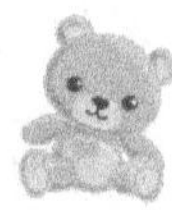
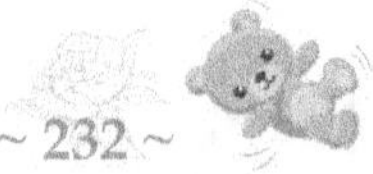
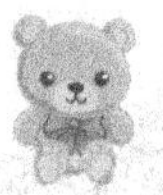

They give me a hand, since it seems to have stopped, but... then I start throwing up; with more diarrhea again, throwing up one more time, and diarrhea, and so on and so forth. I don't know how long it went on for. I'm so tired.

"How long is it going to last, mami? I c-c-can't... I can't take it anymore... I'm in pain and I'm freezing. I don't want it to keep on going, mamita," I tell her in a broken voice, separating every word from the other. I feel like crying for hours, but I don't even have the smallest bit of energy for that.

This whole situation seems endless: toilet, vomit, vomit, toilet, toilet, pee, vomit, vomit, toilet, pee, and on like this, until they give me a bucket to throw up while I'm pooping. Tears fill my eyes. My butt hurts, along with my throat, my belly, my back, my legs, my arms... I want to give up, but my body still feels like throwing out everything ugly it's kept inside. It doesn't give me a break. She tells me that my body is having a quick detox, and since this is happening now, I will feel much better soon. That sounds good, but right now, it's really exhausting.

It stopped! Or, at least, I hope so.

The moment this battle ends, my sleep is heavier than ever. First, they weigh me, and find that I instantly lost three kilograms. Then my mommy and Babulia give me a quick warm shower before carrying me to bed. I think I'm falling asleep in mamita's arms... I will finally get to rest.

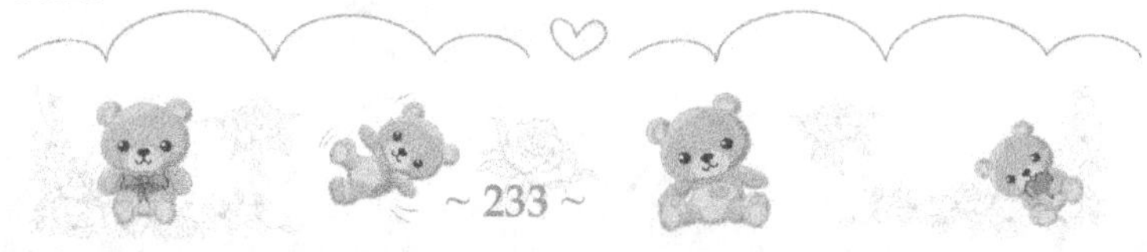

HEALTHY XMAS EVE

I wake up the next day after sleeping for thousands of hours. Although I'm still weak, my pain has yielded, much more so than before. I don't remember the last time I felt like this. I want to make the most of this day, so I better not even look at the bed... today, I'll forget it exists. I'm going to spend some time with my family!

I'm starving, so mamita makes me some delicious juice and a light meal to regain my energy. Klim and my uncle Ilusha are playing PlayStation; they always make hilarious jokes that crack me up, so I didn't think twice about joining the gang. I'm having a great time!

"How do you feel, honey?" mommy asks, approaching me.

"Good, mamita. I feel great!" I answer her and keep playing, killing I don't know who... what is this game about?

The boys have fun with boring things, but even though I don't understand anything about their silly games, they look so excited playing them that they make me laugh out loud. So I'll stay here while there are no girls at home. My cousins Adelina and Melani will be arriving in the evening and we'll play girly games for as long as we want!

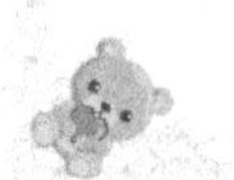
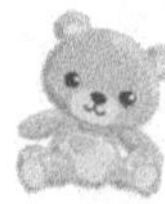
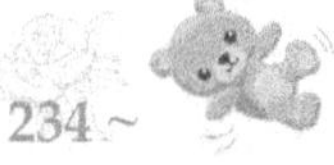
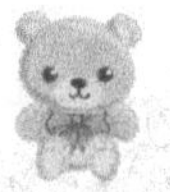

It's Christmas tonight and we're having a delicious vegan dinner – with lots of vegetables, and no meat, milk, or eggs – which mamita taught babulia and my auntie Liubasha.

It's a simple family dinner. We follow the "Caga tio" tradition, as people usually do in Catalonia. It's about a tree trunk with a head and with four legs made of wood. Its back is covered with a red blanket and it has a little red hat – like Santa Claus', but smaller. Children are supposed to hit the poor "Caga tio" with a stick so that he can poop; the funny thing is that his poop is not brown, nor does it smell bad. Instead, it's a bunch of yummy sweets. We smack him with all our strength with a broom, until my uncle Ilusha, who is the strongest in the house, hits him so hard that he breaks the broom stick in half. We burst out laughing, but babulia burst out of the room. I think she's mad at him.

After the beating we gave poor "Caga tio", I still laugh at him because his mouth is drawn with a twisted smile, and his round eyes of different sizes, made from paper scraps, make him look like a clown.

We find all the hidden sweets behind the blanket. This year, we don't have the same candies they usually give us, but small, non-edible gifts and a few exotic fruits. Duuuuull! Anyways, I know that it's much healthier than all the sugar that kept the cancer cells fed; plus, now that I don't eat milk chocolates or dead animals, I feel better.

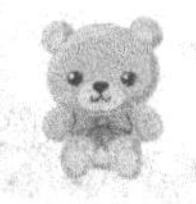 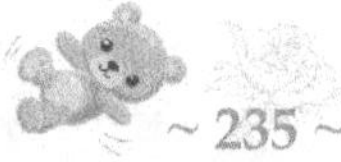 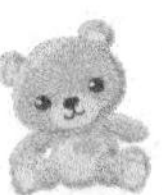 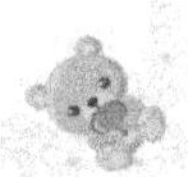

After that terrible night, I've been feeling a little weak, but without any unbearable ache. And I'm not swollen like before, but rather thin like a model.

We spend our Christmas dinner giggling, all reunited, and my pain no longer bothers me as much as it did during these last weeks..

DED MOROZ IN NEW YEAR

We've spent days searching for ingredients and ideas for the party's food, and now New Year's Eve is finally here.

My daily routine remains the same: bathing in seawater, taking medicinal plants, eating organic food, going for walks, and joy... a lot of joy! I feel much better since mamita removed the morphine from my daily intakes. Now my aches generally stay steady at three points on the pain scale, and only go up to six in the evenings.

In Russia, there's an old man who brings winter to the earth. He's dressed up in a long red coat, and carries a huge magic cane with an ice ball on top. People say that Ded Moroz strikes his cane on the ground wherever he walks, covering it with snow.

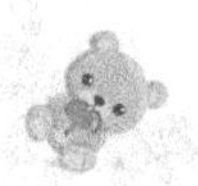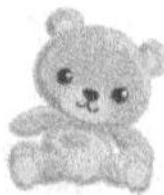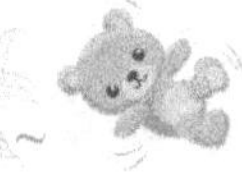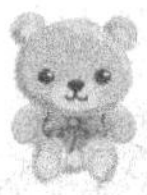

And there's something else – if you touch the ball, you will instantly be frozen. This Russian Santa Claus is always accompanied by his granddaughter Snegurochka. Our family brings together two very different cultures. So our Santa is unique in the world, with a cane, but without Snegurochka.

The main holiday for Russian families is New Year, which is always impatiently awaited. Even though I'm from Russia, I've never been there before. But like my entire family, I follow all their traditions; like the upcoming one: Santa Claus's visit on December 31st. On New Year's Eve, everyone prepares something fun – contests, dances, songs, anything for when he arrives home, and if we don't prepare anything, we make up something along the way since he always stays to have a good time until January 1st.

My cousins prepare some cool dances for the party. Adelina is a very creative and famous gymnast; in fact, she is the best in the world. She always choreographs some nice dance routines for me to perform. There are some that the three of us perform – I mean, her sister Melani, her, and I. When I grow up, I'm going to be just as creative as Adelina, and I'll create lots of dances.

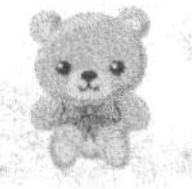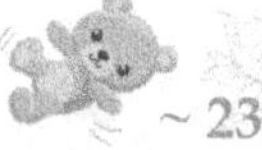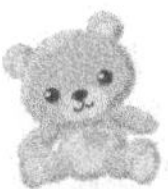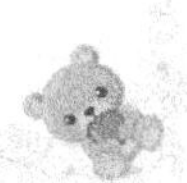

This New Year celebration is crazy! We run around in a hurry; some get busy with preparing dinner, while some others decorate the house or the table. The thing is that everyone keeps busy looking for something, whether it's for glasses and plates of the same color, utensils, pretty napkins... Oh! And we can't forget about the dresses or the pretty clothes for the party! So many things! Everything needs to be ready for dinner. The Christmas tree is the center of attention, but that's already been decorated because it'd been used in Spain on December 25th, and I'd been having a terrible time then. Anyway, it turned out gorgeous without my help.

It smells great in the kitchen. We're all anxious to try the new vegan dishes... Oh!! Oh!! Oh!! And we can't forget about the twelve grapes we eat during the last twelve bells of the year!! We have to calculate carefully so that no one has either more or less. All the Spanish people turn on the same TV channel to follow the tradition, which means we need to keep twelve wishes in mind; since I have many, I count the grapes in my glass several times to make sure that I don't miss a single one. I also try to choose the smallest sizes to eat them quickly because I never get to finish them. That won't happen this time.

The final section of the planning arrives – getting ready. This includes the hair, the pretty dresses, the make-up, the boys wearing their well-ironed shirts with very elegant trousers and shiny shoes; even their thin laces seem to be made of plastic because of how shiny they are.

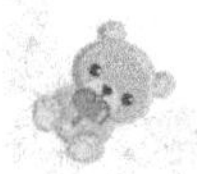
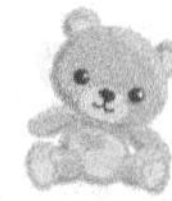
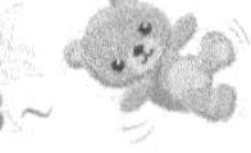

It's eight o'clock in the evening. A few family friends have already started to arrive, so I think we can start our delicious dinner. Let the celebration begin!

The food is tasty… no! No… I'm wrong… it's exquisite! It's completely different though. We usually prepare "pelmenis", white ravioli with minced meat that can never be missed at any Russian party. This version of ours has different colors. It's neither white or wheat flour, but grey with dots, made of spelt and buckwheat flour. Mommy says they have a lot of fiber, which is great for our good gut bacteria; it helps them reproduce faster, and they can protect us from many diseases. We don't stuff vegan pelmenis with meat, but with cabbage and onions. When the cooks make them, they always leave one filled with only dough, and whoever gets it will have good luck all year round. The sour smetana cream was changed to soya or coconut yoghurt. It has an interesting taste, which is a bit strange at first, but you get used to it really fast.

Everyone helps out in the kitchen with the pelmenis because it's a quite an elaborate recipe; besides, since the flour is lighter and not so sticky, it is difficult to make them stick since they are gluten-free, but we try until it comes out right. When I make them, they have different shapes and sizes and they look a bit funny, not like mamita's, which are all the same and perfect.

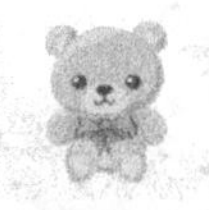 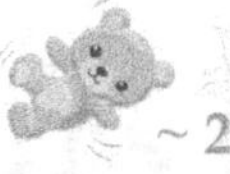 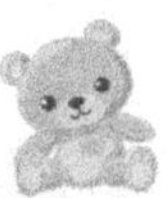 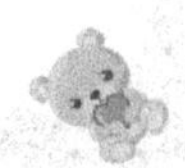

These look a bit odd because they are not white, like before, but they are still delicious. There are also many salads, creams, cheeses, and desserts at the table... And everything is vegan! I know I wasn't completely convinced about this kind of food, but at least I no longer have eczema, or itching – all thanks to my new diet.

We're surrounded by so many different flavors on the table, which looks somewhat new, but is quite tasty. I can't eat much since I'm still recovering, and plus I don't want to repeat the story from a few days ago. My mommy helps me by telling me what I can and can't eat, even though the table is completely vegan, I still have some limits. In fact, I don't even eat much... but my eyes are bigger than my stomach anyways; I could eat each dish with them, but I know I'm too little to even try it. Besides, I don't want to go through another awful night, so I better take it easy. My favorite dish is the Russian carrot salad that has nuts, garlic and mayonnaise. Mommy says she's going to learn how to make it herself so it's much healthier.

This year is not only different because of the food, but also because it's the first time that my brother Pavel is not with us! It's much earlier in the USA since the New Year always comes to Europe first. As our midnight approaches, Pavel Skypes us and stays online on a video call. Watching him through the screen makes me think he isn't alone, and neither are we.

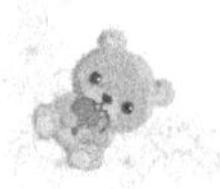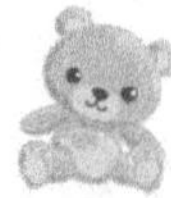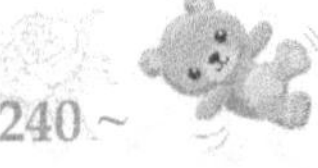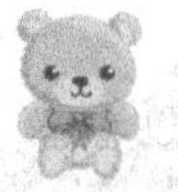

The time has come! The TV clock starts counting down twelve chimes, one for each grape and wish.

Everyone gets to their feet like crazy and starts eating their grapes. I've already written down my wishes on a list so that I don't forget a single one, but the bells are so fast that I'm running out of time.

"Mamita! Mamita, I can't go so fast, I can't!"

"It's alright, baby. Bite only half of each one, that's enough."

Even if I eat only half of them, I don't have time to finish; the bells stop ringing and everyone shouts while my mouth is full of grapes.

"HAPPY NEW YEAR!!!"

We hug and kiss each other, and then we raise our glasses of some non-alcoholic drink... I think it's kombucha or some fresh fruit with water.

How exciting it is to spend holidays with the reunited family!

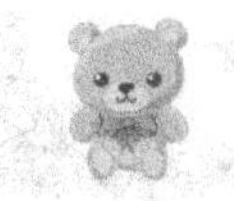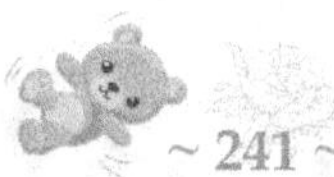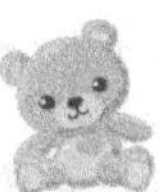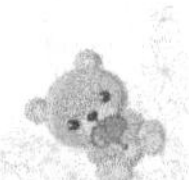

My aches aren't as bad as they used to be. Even when something bothers me, it always stays more or less at the third level on the pain scale, and with how happy I am, it hides in the shadows... even though I know it's there, I'd rather pretend it doesn't exist.

I can't wait for Santa Claus to bring the presents. Honestly, I think it's the most fun part of the party. I love presents! We don't expect much, when mamita suddenly opens the door of babulia's house and shouts, "There's a noise upstairs! Let's find out who it is!"

We go up to the top floor which ends up on the roof. There's a balcony there and we can hear some noises, followed by Santa's voice.

"Ho, ho, ho!"

We keep hearing Santa's laughter, followed by a weird noise as he goes downstairs. My aunt Liubasha and my mom help him drag a couple of bags to the lounge. The first thing Santa does when he arrives is to take a seat.

"I'm so tired! Ugh! I need a glass of water," he says in a very low voice. "Here, I brought you many gifts, but I can only give them to you if you show me something creative."

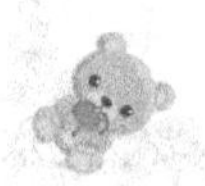
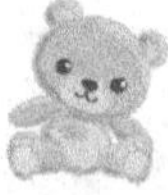
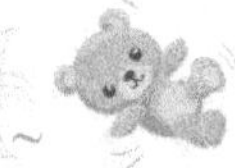
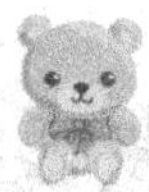

We all take our seats around Santa Claus and watch as he puts his huge hand inside the bag to reach for the first present, and then I hear my name. I'm the first one! Cool! I already have a performance set for him, so I start dancing as soon as Adelina puts on the music; everyone applauds me and I feel like a real superstar. Once I finish, I sit on his knees to give him a kiss, then I hug him tight and get my present. Actually, I receive lots of them throughout the party, but I don't have enough shows prepared... What should I do? I'll make something up. Maybe I could sit on a split or do the bridge, which comes out perfectly. Every time I do something that includes bending my head down, I get dizzy, but I want to have fun with my family because this party only happens once a year. When I run out of ideas, they sing with me, or create meaningless fun dances, and we laugh endlessly. There are many gifts for everyone, so they better think of some creative things to do.

The last part of the party is the best – Santa's gift. With so many pillows wrapped under the suit, that seems like a big belly, it's very funny to see him dancing to rap... seriously, his belly is so big that it jiggles and almost escapes him, so we burst out laughing. Mommy and auntie Liubasha did a great job organizing everything. Thanks to them, no one was left without a gift and we all had a great time together.

During the final show with my cousins Adelina and Melani, everyone applauds joyfully and we'd like to choreograph other dances in the future. It's the greatest thing!

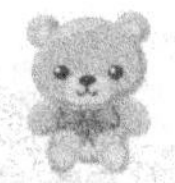 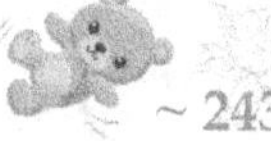 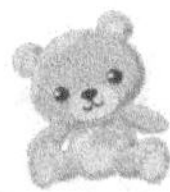 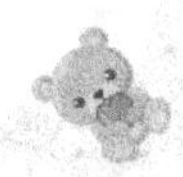

We usually go to bed at six in the morning because everyone has so much energy that we have to keep playing and goofing around. However, this New Year is shorter for me than for the others. I don't know what time they went to bed, but I fall asleep much earlier because I'm bushed. Nonetheless, I'm happy about the great day we had though.

On January 1st, 2015, we wake up super late, but there are more surprises awaiting us. So we shake off the laziness right away and run to get our special gifts. Every year, we find huge, red Christmas stockings with our names on them, and the best is yet to come – they're full of sweets that we could eat for months! Mine is a bit flattened, since it doesn't have as many candies and chocolates as the previous years, but has a variety of fruits, and a few yummy things from the organic shop. Honestly, I'm in love with my first healthy christmas stocking. Mommy called it "Bye Bye Cancer". Now you know where I got the inspiration for this book's title.

After taking lots of family photos with our presents, we sit on the floor to take everything out of our stockings, put it between our legs so that it doesn't get mixed up with the others', and study every single thing we got this year. We show each other the sweets, negotiate them and exchange whatever we don't like… and if we don't get a proper deal, we give it away. Although I can't do much swapping, I enjoy sharing quite a lot.

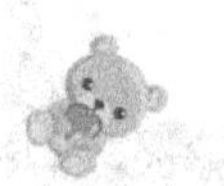
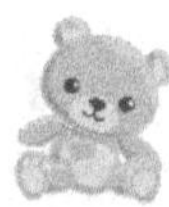
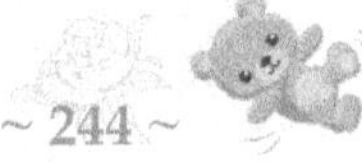
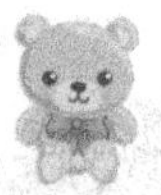

We have a great time, and even more so because I've never felt better; but it's time to go home. We pack our bags and buy things that we can't find in Ireland, especially whatever's missing for my natural treatment. Then my daddy takes us to Barcelona's airport and the holidays are over! We're on our way home. I will never forget these holidays!

NEW AIRS IN CHARLESTOWN

We arrive in Charlestown. My old medicine box is still here and just seeing it makes me sick. So we immediately put them away, and they're only going to be brought out when the Hospice group come to visit. As soon as they resume the visits, they ask me how my trip went and how I felt during the holidays, but I just tell them I feel the same and that there's not really much more I can say. Although the plants and supplements I'm taking seem to be working, mommy told me it's a secret, so I keep my mouth shut; she shows the doctors the medicine box, telling them that we aren't missing anything, and they leave without getting suspicious. The truth is that I have my energy back, and I feel great about restarting our normal daily routine… like going to school and stuff, you know?

Everyone is surprised by my change, especially because of how skinny I got; Sue and Olga are always asking me how I'm doing, offering mommy to help us with whatever we need. They are really good people.

Now I even have some more friends at school. We hang out, and go together to a 12 year old's disco in a village called Banada! It's great to spend some time with my friends. It makes me feel like an adult since mamita lets me go.

We've spent four months following this new lifestyle, doing lots of different things like the fruit-days, where we eat tons of the same fruit for the whole day. I used to hate oranges before – not to mention orange juice. I could never drink it, but now I find them so delicious... It's my favorite fruit-day! I love pineapple too, though, once we ate it nonstop for three days in a row, I didn't even want to see it anymore after a certain point since my tongue got irritated from so much acidity. The apple day is the easiest because they last pretty well. I eat and eat and it seems like I haven't even taken a single bite; mommy says I can eat their seeds because they attack cancer cells with their vitamin B17, which are also called amygdalin. That's the reason why they are so bitter. The apricots' seeds are the same way, and also bad-tasting. I don't like them at all and sometimes they even paralyze my mouth. Still, mommy says I must eat them, so I do.

Everything is easier when it's fasting day because we don't have to worry about food – just water, tons of water.

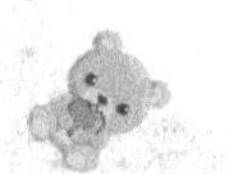
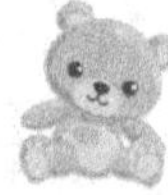
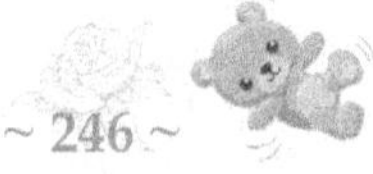
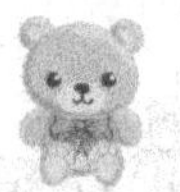

Mami started studying nutrition at a school. Sometimes she goes to Madrid for a few days and babulia comes to watch after us. Though we are already grown up, we can't stay home alone. Olga gives us a hand whenever my granny can't, and even Andrés take care of us from time to time. He always has time to play on the PlayStation with me. There are thousands of games, but the best ones are Shrek and a racing car one that my brothers had. We have a lot of fun together!

One day, mommy tells the Hospice's group that we don't need their support anymore, which caught them by surprise. They didn't understand what was happening. As soon as they left the house, mommy and I jump up and down with excitement, laughing at our mischief. We finally got rid of them!

"It isn't time to say anything to anyone. Let's keep this to ourselves for now, dóchenka."

Mami is discovering more and more things. She tells me that we have to go on like this for at least six more months.

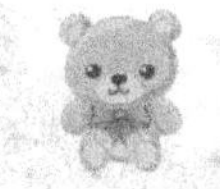 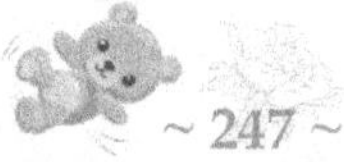 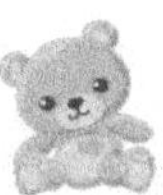 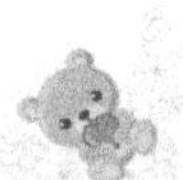

It's April, 2015, and I really want to ride a bike. I have no idea where this desire came from, but I feel like it's time. So I take Klim's to the street, which is a bit heavy for learning, but also low enough that I can just balance myself with my feet if I feel like I'm going to fall. Mommy sends my brother to give me a hand as soon as she realizes what I'm doing, but I don't want any help. I want to do it myself. Even so, he keeps an eye on me.

After many tries, suddenly, the bicycle starts responding to what I command... or rather, because of the pedaling, it starts moving slowly, and I don't fall down. I think the hardest thing about riding a bike is controlling the shaky handlebar. It isn't as stable as I would like. Anyway, I'm proud of myself and feel like I'm flying.

"Mom!! Mommy!!! Katerina is riding the bike!!! Quick!!! Quick mom!!" I hear Klim's voice behind me, and it makes me feel prouder somehow.

"One more time, dóchenka!! Do it again!! You're doing it great!!" I repeat the same steps over and over again.

This day, I've learned how to ride a bike, and I know it took me a long time, but as Klim always tells me "better late than never".

One day, we go to do the MRI in Dublin. Dr. Kapra is impressed with the results, and even more so with my sudden recovery.

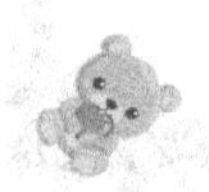 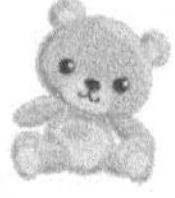 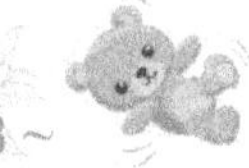 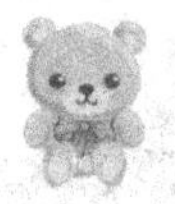

"I find Katerina perfect, wow! I'm very surprised. What have you done, mom?"

My mommy starts telling him our secret – about the new diet, the new medicinal plants supplements... but suddenly the doctor interrupts her.

"That's it, mom, no more."

As soon as we leave his office mamita says, "It's weird that he didn't want to hear everything we did... I just started to tell him... Don't you think it's weird that he wasn't interested?"

Maybe he didn't believe her, or just didn't want to know…whatever. The important thing is that I feel better. Great, I'd say. I no longer remember the hard months I went through, nor do I want to; and I wouldn't wish that on anyone, least of all a child! I had to be very, very strong to get through it.

The year went by quickly with no signs of my illness, no aches, no eczemas. I have nothing but an incredible amount of energy and desire to do things I've never done before. I love my new diet, by the way, and mamita is now a master in the kitchen. I'm also learning to make dishes as delicious as hers. Actually, we prepare them together very often. Our cookbook already has thousands of recipes. We haven't had time to try them all, of course, but the fridge is full of healthy food that we can experiment with.

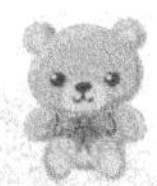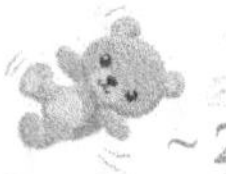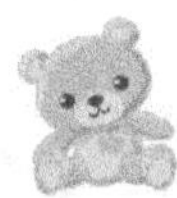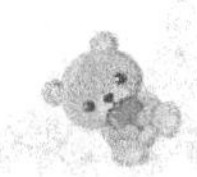

The school has been going great too. I found out that I'm a very creative person, and have become an expert in making school projects. I don't intend to brag, but they're amazing! The kids in my class even wait impatiently to see what I can do. Since they know I'm always carrying something new and interesting, they surround me and ask me to take the wrapping off, and are always shocked when I show them what I've done.

"WOOOW! How did you do it, Kate? It's very nice!" They ask me thousands of questions.

Some classmates try to make similar things, but I am an expert. They struggle with trying to get similar results, but can't seem to quite get there; besides, for each new school project, I come up with even wilder ideas, whether they are posters or something else in 3D... no one ever beat me.

Thus, without realizing it, without being tied to doctors or hospitals, the summer of 2015 finally arrives. Klim and I are going to spend our vacations in Spain, but this time, we will enjoy them like never before because there will be no treatments or suffering – just family and friends! I'll even spend a few days with my daddy and my other brother, Robin. I'm so happy to feel good again! It's amazing to leave the bad times behind!

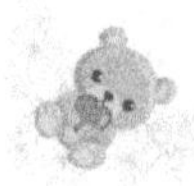
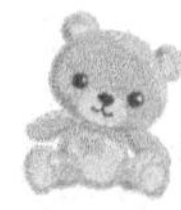
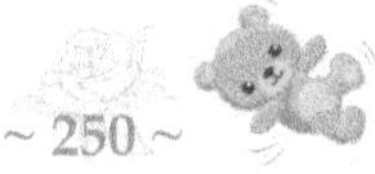
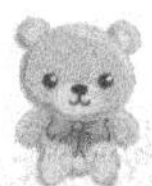

For the whole summer, I attend to a camp from morning until noon, where I participate in many great activities, like swimming, and the one I love the most – rhythmic gymnastics; in Charlestown, they only have boxing and Gaelic, which is a form of soccer. I don't like any of those sports, so I better practice my favorites here, every day, during June.

After a few days at babulia's house, mamita goes to Los Angeles, USA, where she is supposed to get together with Pavel. It has been a year since he left, and we all miss him like crazy; lucky mommy for having the chance to spend summer with him. By the way, she even made a new friend there. His name is Thomas, and he told her he would come meet us in October.

Our vacations are over and we're going back to Ireland to continue our school year. This is the last one for Klim, who is also doing the same paperwork and exams as Pavel because he wants to study at a university in the USA too. Mamita still hasn't decided if we'll go back to Spain, or if we'll move to a smaller apartment in Dublin. I honestly don't care. I'd go anywhere, as long as mami and I are together.

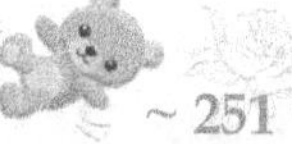
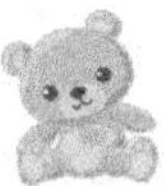
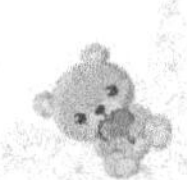

October reaches us in a flash. Thomas is already here! Mamita says he will stay with us for three weeks and also tells us he's a vegan. Great! I'd never met anyone with our lifestyle before. Besides, he knows a lot about technology… that's cool. We like him, and I think we're already friends. One day, mommy and Thomas go to Belfast for a visit, but Klim and I can't go because we have school. However, on weekends, we always show Tommy the most beautiful places we know in this country. Anyway, once they get back, Klim and I are called to gather in the kitchen. I heard it's about some good news, so we are anxious... what will it be? At the moment, I only see their cheerful faces.

"Klim and Katerina… Thomas and I got engaged, and we're getting married soon!" They show us the beautiful rings they bought in Belfast.

What?! How?! I don't understand anything... Is mommy going to get married?! We immediately jump with joy, happy for them.

"Wow!! Congratulations!! How nice, mom, congratulations!!" we say, giving them both kisses.

So, my mommy's getting married... WOW! The lovebirds told us we're going to move to the USA when the school year ends, but first, there are some procedures to be taken care of.

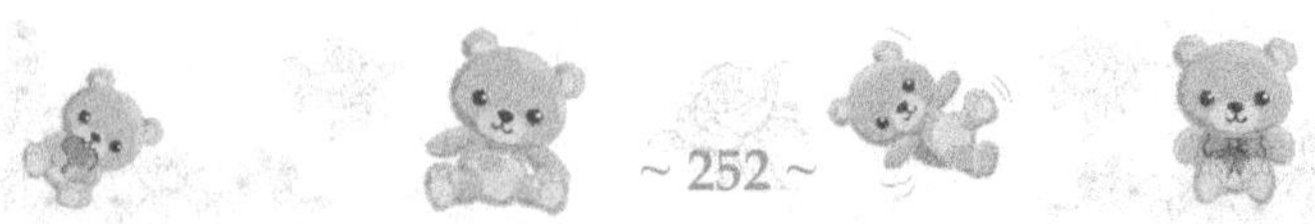

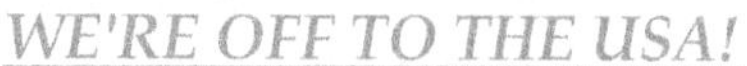

WE'RE OFF TO THE USA!

My second year in secondary school will be over soon, and I'll be starting the freshman year in the USA. It's very exciting! Klim is applying for his student visa, so he won't leave with us. He has to finish up his exams first, and then travel as a student.

Once his three-week visit got over, Thomas left for the USA, but came back to us right away. The family is complete now; we live together, and we're waiting for these four months to pass quickly so that we can continue with our plans at the end of my school year.

On the last day of school, our teacher congratulates me, and announces that I'm moving to the USA; my cooking classmates prepare a chocolate vegan cake that says "Bon Voyage Kate" for me. It's my fasting day, but seeing how nice and good-tasting the cake looks, I've decided to change it to the next day. My aides give me a beautiful necklace with my name on it, and a good-bye letter signed by all my friends. It's a very special day. We even go to the soccer field together to take some pics and I was right in the middle of them.

We are ready for the trip, and Klim is staying behind, as we agreed; he still has a month left before his final exams and graduation. Babulia, Olga and Andrés, will give him a hand from time to time, but he is a big boy now.

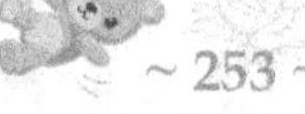

We know he can take care of himself. All our things will be staying here in Ireland – the furniture, the clothes, and the car. Andres will come for my brother when it's time, and he will take him in our car to Spain, from where Klim will travel to the USA, with my granny and Liubasha, as they are all coming to mamita and Thomas' wedding..

WE'RE ALMOST READY!

It's June 5th, 2016, the day of our trip to the USA. As the flight has been scheduled very early in the morning, we have to spend the night in Dublin. After a long journey, including a transfer in Boston, we land at our final destination: San Diego. Yoo-hoo! I'm so excited about living in a new country, and meeting new people and kids my age!

A cab drops us off at our new house, and I'm impressed the moment I see it. It's beautiful! The best thing about it is that we have the Pacific Ocean so close that we can look at it from our window; I even decided to take some surfing lessons. For now, I can't really stand upright on the board, but I still enjoy it. Mommy, and Thomas also have a good time with me at the beach from time to time, and I help them with their wedding planning.

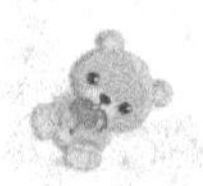 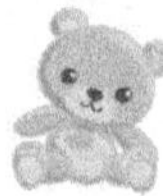 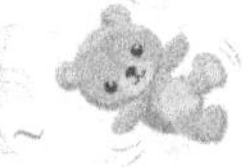 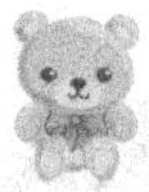

The whole family will be coming out in August and we'll be together again. Pável is studying in Northern California, about 500 miles from us, but it's much closer than before. It's been two years since I last saw him, and I can't wait to hug him.

My auntie Liubasha, Babulia, and Klim arrive first. I don't know how he managed to stay all alone in Ireland, but it seems that he survived because he's here now. Granny says that he kept falling asleep in every corner of the airport, poor thing; with so many exams, he must've been super stressed.

A couple of days go by, and we are all waiting for Pavel to arrive – he's actually the only one missing. We haven't seen him om a long time, so we refuse to go to bed… I mean, it's our reunion! When we finally hear the door, we immediately run to welcome him. I'm the first one to give him a lot of kisses and a huge hug. At that moment, I realize that Pavel is not the same as I remember him: he's become a tall and strong man. I can't believe my brother is already with us! We all cry tears of happiness, wanting to hug him tight, but there are too many of us, and he is only one. So we all jump into bed squeezing him, without letting him go, not even for a little bit. It's an emotional moment; there's so much joy that it's too difficult to express with words what I'm feeling.

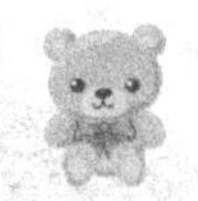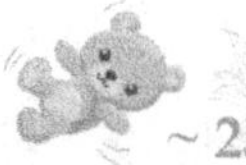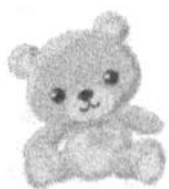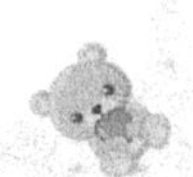

One day before the wedding, we head out to buy whatever we are still missing. We don't really find what we were looking for, except for mamita's shoes. Plus, we girls take advantage of the afternoon to go get manicures and pedicures at the spa, so we have fewer things to do tomorrow.

At night, we decorate the car with beautiful white flowers. What a benefit that our car is also white, because it came out perfect! It's my first time doing this kind of décor, but I love it. I inflate lots of balloons, and paint a sign that says "Just married", but that's for the after-wedding. Oh gosh! How am I supposed to calm down if my mommy gets married tomorrow? TOMORROW!

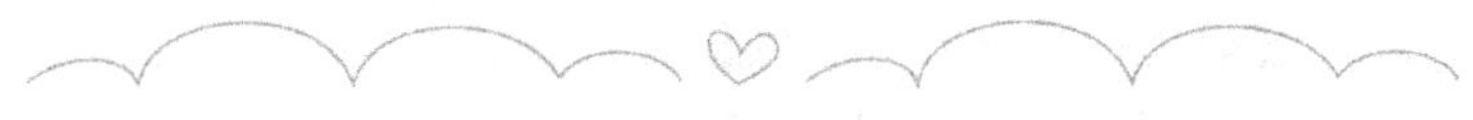

THE WEDDING!

It's August 10th, 2016, the most expected day: mamita's wedding. We wake up very early so we'd have enough time to get ready, to style our hair, do our make-up, wearing our beautiful dresses. We need to be at Coronado Island at two in the afternoon.

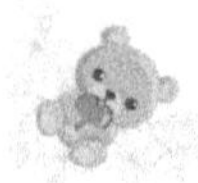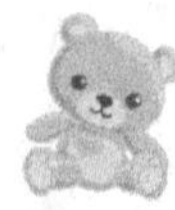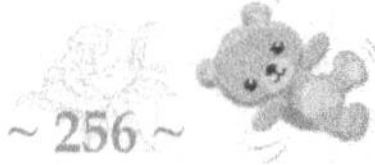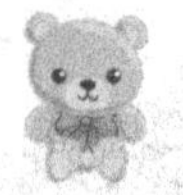

The boys' preparation is easier – they just have to wear the clothes that my mommy ironed and hung for them on the closet doors. My brothers and I will be wearing matching clothes since their shirts are turquoise, just like my dress. They wear white pants, shoes and hats, while Thomas is wearing a white shirt and pants. It looks like my mom will marry a prince! It's like she is living one of those Princesses stories.

We girls have a lot to do, running around up and down the stairs… there's always one thing or another missing and time flies by! My mommy wears her long white wedding dress. It's a Hawaiian styled dress with a flower on one side and a bow on the back. Her hair is decorated with a shiny tiara and a short veil down the back. She looks like a girl in her twenties. I'd say like a princess, but that's saying too little; she's quite a queen!

I'll be going to the ceremony by car with Liubasha and babulia a bit earlier. Pavel will be the bride and groom's driver, who will be sitting in the back seat, while Klim will escort them in the co-pilot's seat.

There are many white chairs arranged neatly for the ceremony, the arch has been decorated with flowers, and the sea behind makes everything look even more gorgeous. Many of the guests have arrived and most of them are Tommy's relatives, which is normal since they all live here. On mommy's side, there aren't many of us – it's just my babulia, Liubasha, Pavel, Klim, a friend of mommy's named Irina, who lives in California, and me.

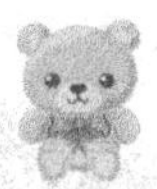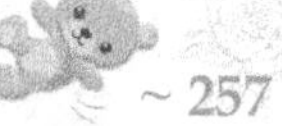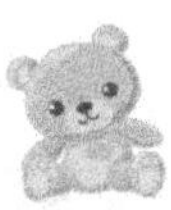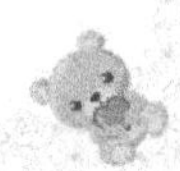

When their car arrives, Pavel and Klim get out first and open their doors on both sides, such gentlemen! At that moment, the wedding music starts playing. Mommy and Thomas walk together to the arch. They look so happy I think I'm about to cry. After some words, they finally say "YES, I DO." That's it! They're married!

We take thousands of pictures all together before heading to the gala room. There's music, lights, and a beautiful table. It's time for the bride and groom to dance!

It's also time to present the surprise I've prepared for the guests. The bride and groom start their romantic dance, but suddenly some lively music plays. They shrug their shoulders without understanding what is happening, and then a few of Thomas and mami's family members get up to dance. At first, the guests looked a bit worried. They didn't even move a finger, but as soon as they noticed that the "dancers" followed the same steps, along with my mommy and Thomas, they started laughing out loud while applauding non-stop. Then the same romantic music starts playing as before, and we quickly leave the stage for the bride and groom to finish their first-dance. We practiced during the whole summer, but it was worth the effort. The performance came out perfect, and everybody liked it. I'm proud to have been the choreographer!

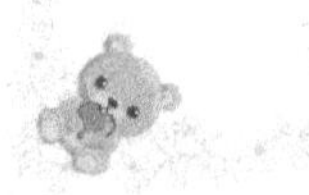 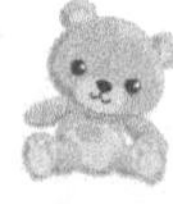 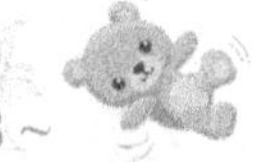 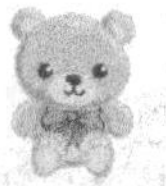

The catering service cooked a Mexican style wedding dinner, completely vegan, of course, and even the cake was made with healthy ingredients. Even though not everyone here shares this lifestyle, all of the guests seem to love the food. None of them realize it was vegan, so they were very surprised. The party was a lot of fun!

At sunset, once the celebration is over, we put up the little sign behind the car and it's time for the newlyweds to leave. Ugh! I think I'm done with responsibilities... for now!.

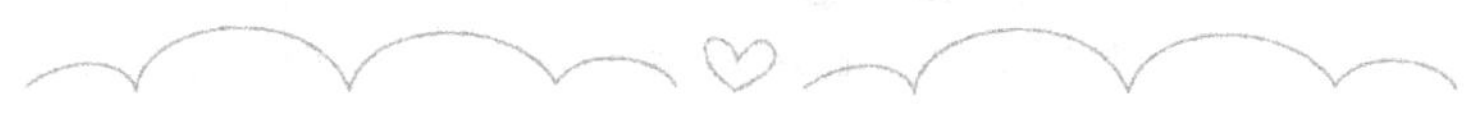

MY NEW HIGH SCHOOL

I'm very nervous because I'll soon be starting my first year at the new school. Everyone here speaks English and luckily, I've already learned it. My accent is really different from the rest though since mine is Irish, and it shows.

I've finally joined Point Loma High School, which is about twenty times bigger than Ireland's – it even looks like a university. It's huge! At first, I get confused with some papers I'm given at the administration office. They have some weird numbers like A102 or G401, I guess they're the subjects? Plus, there's a lot of walking to do, from one classroom to another, which always makes me late, and teachers sent an SMS to mommy warning her about my absence.

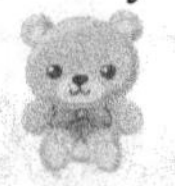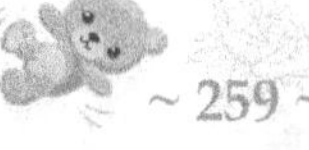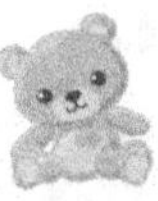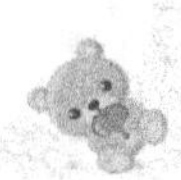

It's a bit complicated, but I'll get used to it...Eventually!

Here, there are many children from different countries, not like in Ireland where I only studied with natives. There are many students from Poland, and some others from China. I feel very happy since I make many friends right from the very first day. Bit by bit, I've been introducing myself to a new community that, honestly, I like very much.

After spending a whole month with us, babulia, and Liubasha must go back to Spain. Having them here was great. I liked taking them to all the beautiful places, but I think it's time to start our daily life in San Diego. Pavel must continue his studies in the East Bay area. This will be his last year of college, and since he's advanced a year, he will be finishing his studies very soon. Klim will be joining San Marcos University, which is an hour away from home, so mamita and Thomas are looking for a comfortable place for him to stay near the campus.

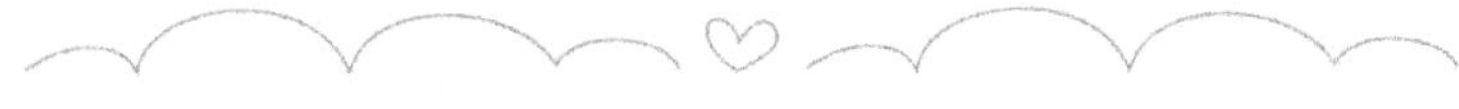

MOMMY'S BOOK

Mamita has been thinking, for a long time, about sharing our story with many people. I find it great and I always encouraged her to write about my cancer, but for some reason she hasn't started yet.

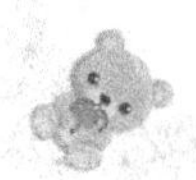
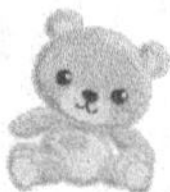
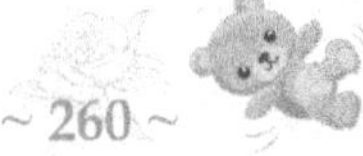
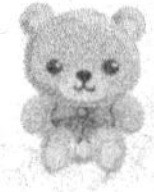

"Dóchenka, you know... I want to write a book. I've already told you several times..."

"Yes mamita, I know. You should write it!"

"Before I do it, I need to tell you something. In my book, I want to write something I haven't told you about and I think it's time for you to know."

"Sure, mami, tell me. What is it?" I'm anxious to know what she's talking about. I don't know if it's in a good or a bad way.

"It's about your cancer, and everything we've been through, especially the last morphine treatment you were taking and the Hospice care. Do you remember?"

"Of course, I remember, mamita. I wish I didn't though... we had an awful time then."

"The truth is... hospice care is a special help for people with very serious illnesses, but when I say serious, I mean it. It's more for people who have no way out."

"I don't understand, mami. What do you mean?"

"When people are prescribed Hospice care, it's because they're so sick there's no hope for a long life. The morphine treatment you were taking had no curative effect per se; it would simply reduce your aches."

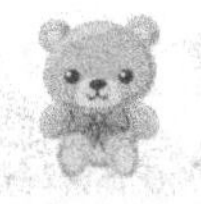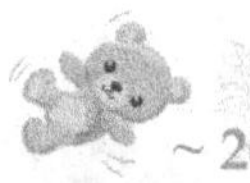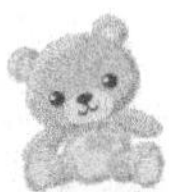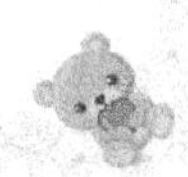

She takes a short pause, and then continues, "It didn't help you much, did it? It turns out that the doctors, before admitting you to the Castlebar's hospital, had already condemned you to your... death bed. They gave you only about... five months to live, dóchenka. They said you wouldn't last much longer."

Suddenly, a mixture of emotions and memories crashed inside my mind, along with a weird sound in my head. Mommy doesn't even let me react and continues right away.

"It wasn't true, dóchenka, it wasn't true what they said. Because we discovered another way so we could save you... just in time. We were able to cheat death, sweetheart."

"But... mamita... Why?" That's all I could say, with trembling lips, while my eyes are so full of tears that I can barely hold them in.

It's hard for me to imagine what she is saying.

"We left everything behind, baby. Everything is in the past. You are safe now, honey, we are safe! There's no more danger in your life."

She hugs me tightly and we break into tears. "I'm telling you this now because I want to write this book and tell the story exactly as it happened. I can't write it without you knowing. You agree, honey?"

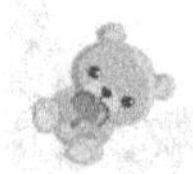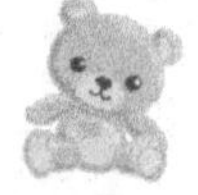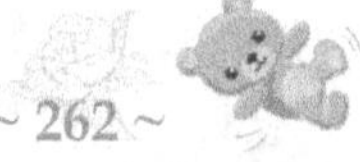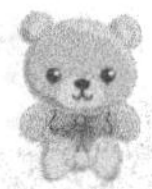

"Yes, mamita, of course, do it... so that people know our story."

I'm trying to analyze what she just told me, but my tears are bigger than my eyes. It took me several days to understand why the doctors gave me only five months of life.

I just turned 14 and I understand many more things now. Most of the time, I repeat in my head, over and over again, what my mom had told me.

"It's all in the past, baby. You are a healthy and strong girl... actually, the strongest girl on the planet," she tells me in her sweet voice, whenever I ask her about it.

At the moment, I let it go, but after a few days...

"Was I really going to die, mamita? Really?"

"Of course not, dóchenka!! I'm your mother, and I'm right by your side so that nothing bad ever happens to you, I'm here to protect you. That's what I did, or rather... we did it together, right? I wouldn't let anything harm you, baby girl."

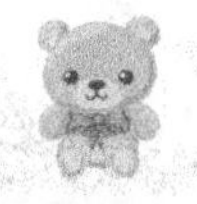 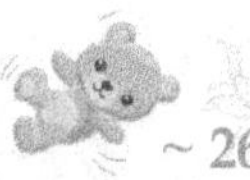 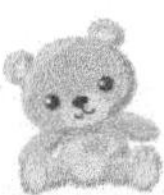 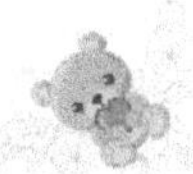

I spent some time going through an acceptance process. I was only able to calm down after hearing, my mommy say "Everything's okay now", a million times, with such confidence that I kick that idea out of my head. I decided to continue to enjoy my life, as healthy as I am. That's what matters now. Thanks to my mommy! As soon as I understood that clearly, a new desire showed up in my mind: to write my own book, telling our story from my experience.

My mommy would write one focusing on her view, and her feelings. She would talk about her struggles to save my life. I decided to write mine with the same story, but as seen through my own eyes, with everything I've lived in my own skin. The feelings and thoughts of the six-year-old little girl that I was, and who knew nothing of this world.

Here I am, remembering every moment, asking my family for help reconstruct the past, and put everything on paper. It isn't easy, but I did my best to analyze everything with full awareness and an understanding of reality.

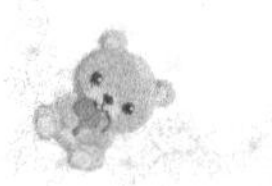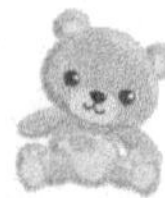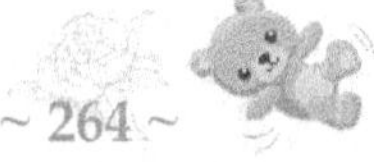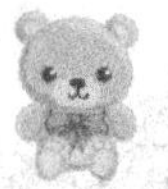

My mom, Liudmila Gersten, has already published her book entitled "Y Katerina bailó con la muerte", which has a second edition named: "Bye-Bye Cancer". When my book comes out, hers will surely be around the world, and how couldn't it? She did a great job, even writing in three languages (Spanish, English and Russian) so that it reaches a wider audience. That's the way I want to do it. The best thing about publishing both her perspective and mine, is so that some parts of the story can be understood much better.

I'm reaching the end of my book at 16 years old. I hope to complete the processes of preparation, layout, design and publication quickly. How exciting! I can't wait for you to read about what we went through.

Mommy, Thomas, and I came to Costa Rica for our summer holidays, and we're having a great time; we're surrounded by wild animals... I don't even know what some of them are. I'm finishing these last few pages, sitting on a wooden bench under a roof made of palm leaves in Mono Congo, an open to nature coffee shop in front of the Barú River. The sea behind me makes a magical and hypnotizing sound. Besides, the sunset here is gorgeous and it has so many beautiful colors that relaxes me. It allows me to focus and get even more inspired to keep writing... it's a tropical paradise. I just write and watch the landscape, enjoying the moment.

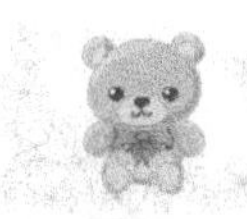
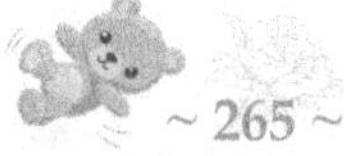
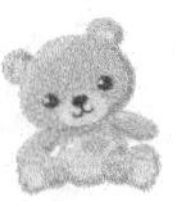
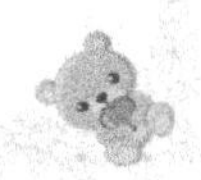

There is no one in the establishment at this moment because it's six o'clock in the afternoon and they'd already closed an hour ago. But since they have a Wi-Fi connection, I continue writing. Lucky that they don't kick us out! You can't imagine the pleasure I feel right now. Mommy and Thomas don't rush me either – quite the opposite really. They wait for me patiently, while they do their things. Mommy is sitting next to me, posting about the Costa Rica trip on her Instagram and Thomas is discussing something about a land we will most likely buy in Puerto Viejo. So, I got to the end of my book, which seemed endless. I made it! But don't worry, my life is going to continue with many more adventures and emotions.

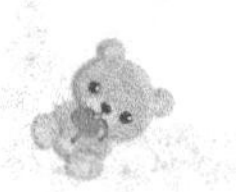
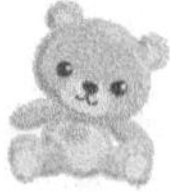
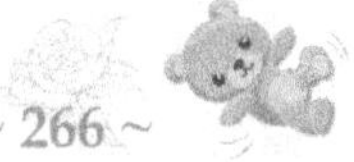
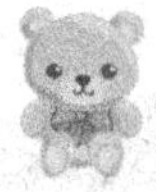

WEIRD VOCABULARY IN MY BOOK

- **BABULIA** — BABULIA (RUSSIAN) - GRANDMOTHER.

- **DÓCHENKA / DOCHKA (RUSSIAN)** — DAUGHTER (IN MINIATURE), DAUGHTER.

- **MÁMACHKA (RUSSIAN)** — MOMMY.

- **VNÚCHENKA (RUSSIAN)** — NIETECITA.

- **SOLNISHKO MAIO (RUSSIAN)** — MY LITTLE SUNSHINE.

- **PRIVET, MOI DOROGIE VNUCHATA! (RUSSIAN)** — HELLO, MY DEAR GRANDCHILDREN.

- **SINOCHKI (RUSSIAN)** — CHILDREN.

- **SMETANA (RUSSIAN)** — SOFT TEXTURED SOUR CREAM, WITH AN ACIDIC TASTE.

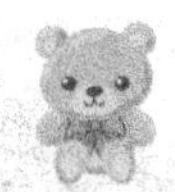 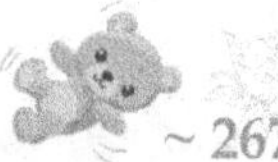 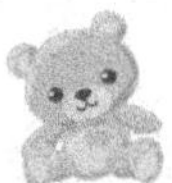 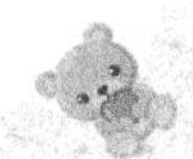

- **PIROZHKÍ (RUSSIAN)** — TYPICAL RUSSIAN EMPANADAS FILLED WITH MINCED MEAT AND ONION, OR SHREDDED CARROTS WITH SUGAR AND BUTTER, OR CABBAGE WITH CARAMELIZED ONIONS OR MASHED POTATOES. THIS IS VERY TYPICAL IN RUSSIA.

- **PELMENI (RUSSIAN)** — FESTIVE DISH IN RUSSIA SIMILAR TO RAVIOLI, BUT ALMOST ALL THE TIME THEY ARE MADE BY HAND FILLED WITH EITHER MINCED MEAT AND ONION OR CABBAGE AND ONION. A FESTIVE DISH IN RUSSIA.

- **MEDOVIK (RUSSIAN)** — RUSSIAN HONEY CAKE WITH EIGHT (8) LAYERS AND CREAM BETWEEN THEM.

- **PÓ DELAM (RUSSIAN)** — SETTLE SOME MATTERS.

- **PÓSOH (RUSSIAN)** — RUSSIAN SANTA CLAUS' LONG WALKING STICK.

- **DED MOROZ (RUSSIAN)** — SANTA CLAUS.

- **YA ZDES SÓLNICHKO (RUSSIAN)** — I'M HERE, SUNSHINE.

- **KEIT (ENGLISH), KATUSHA (RUSSIAN) KATERINA, EKATERINA** — DIFFERENT LOVELY WAYS OF SAYING MY NAME.

- **YAYA (SPANISH)** — THAT'S WHAT PEOPLE CALL MY GRANNY IN BARCELONA.

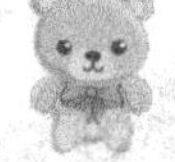

- **CALMANTES (SPANISH)** — THESE ARE THE FAMOUS "PAINKILLERS".

- **MAKE-A-WISH (ENGLISH)** — NON-PROFIT COMPANY THAT GIVES THE CHANCE OF FULFILLING WISHES TO CHILDREN WHO HAVE LIFE-THREATENING MEDICAL CONDITIONS.

- **MAAGIC FLIGHT** — AMERICAN AIRLINES ASSOCIATION, HENCE THE DOUBLE AA. PROVIDES CHILDREN MAGICAL EXPERIENCES DURING THEIR FLIGHTS.

- **MAGIC KINGDOM** — PARK LOCATED AT WALT DISNEY WORLD RESORT IN LAKE BUENA VISTA, ORLANDO.

- **GIVE KIDS THE WORLD** — NON-PROFIT COMPLEX IN KISSIMMEE, FLORIDA, THAT PROVIDES LODGING IN THE MAGIC KINGDOM FOR CRITICALLY ILL CHILDREN AND THEIR FAMILIES

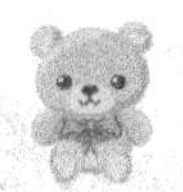 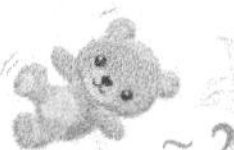 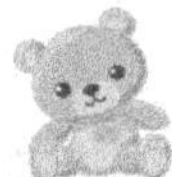 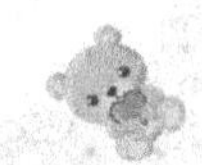